Prescription: Murder

Over His Dead Body
&
A "C" Change

Two Novellas in the Ham Marks, MD,
Murder-Mystery Series

WILLIAM H. SIMON, MD

iUniverse, Inc.
Bloomington

Prescription: Murder

iUniverse books may be ordered through booksellers or by contacting:

iUniverse
1663 Liberty Drive
Bloomington, IN 47403
www.iuniverse.com
1-800-Authors (1-800-288-4677)

ISBN: 978-1-4697-8828-9 (sc)
ISBN: 978-1-4759-1771-0 (ebk)

Printed in the United States of America

iUniverse rev. date: 05/21/2012

Author's Note

Prescription Murder contains the first two books in the Ham Marks, MD, murder-mystery series.

The first novella, *Over His Dead Body*, introduces Ham Marks, MD, a forensic orthopedic surgeon, and follows his actions and mishaps as he unravels the hospital-based murder of a malpractice lawyer.

The second novella, *A "C" Change*, provides even greater insight into the thought processes of Dr. Marks as he and his wife, Ruth, take what they think will be an enjoyable Mediterranean cruise. During the trip, Ham describes a number of death-defying incidents that occur to him as he tries, unsuccessfully, to prevent the murder of a Bulgarian medical colleague who has invented a fabulous skin cream that is potentially worth billions to its owner.

A "C" Change also introduces Ham's alter ego—a Bulgarian secret service agent who, along with Ham's friend, an FBI agent, saves Ham's life in this murderous adventure.

All the characters named in these two books are fictitious. Any resemblance to people alive or dead is purely coincidental.

Contents

OVER HIS DEAD BODY

A "C" CHANGE

CHAPTER 1

CARPE DIEM

Take advantage of the day

The office door opened and a large man entered. He was six feet three and weighed around 230 pounds. He was big but not menacing. More huggable—like a large teddy bear. And he was slightly balding and stoop-shouldered.

The office door opened into a large waiting room of his medical practice. It had about twenty leather and wood chairs, oriental rugs on the floor and on the wall, and enlarged and framed photographs of many of the exotic lands the doctor and his wife had visited in the past twenty years. To his left was a reception desk, and beyond that was the business office where four white-coated women worked.

"Carpe diem," the man said.

But this wasn't a foreign land. And it certainly wasn't the land where this language was spoken. This was on Seventeenth Street, in the middle of Philadelphia, and he was speaking ancient Latin, the language of long-dead Romans. The four ladies in white replied chorus-like, "Good morning, Dr. Marks."

They had no idea what he had said to them. (Actually he had said in the other language, "Seize the day," a phrase that for him meant "Have a good day.") But they were so used to this man greeting them each morning with a Latin salutation that they continued on with their work as if it were an everyday occurrence—which it was for them!

The man was Ham Marks, MD, a fellow of the American College of Surgeons. He was sixty-three years old, and since he had recently given up an active surgical practice—he'd told his wife, "Leave it to the younger guys with less arthritis in their fingers"—most of his peers considered him a forensic orthopedist. Forensic, in this case, not referring to a CSI type but rather a trained orthopedic surgeon whose job was to figure out, by using his knowledge of anatomy, pathology, and physiology as well as his clinical and research knowledge of the musculoskeletal system, just what caused what. Did that fall down the steps at work cause the disintegration of the hip joint that necessitated a total-hip replacement? Or was it inevitable? Did that automobile accident, with its attendant "whiplash," cause the herniated disc? Or was it a degenerative condition that was just brought to light because of an investigation of neck pain? These were questions that fell into the realm of the medico-legal aspects of orthopedics, where money was involved—lots and lots of money.

The Latin thing, that was another story. Ham's mother had been a classicist, a teacher of ancient Latin and Greek. She had whimsically (or perhaps out of professional pride) christened him Homer Alcibiades Marks in order to connect him indelibly with two of her ancient heroes.

Times being what they were, Homer Alcibiades Marks quickly became Ham Marks, a nickname that permanently obscured the full name's ancient provenance through grade school, high school, Princeton University, Harvard Medical School, and beyond.

Ham moved down a short hall and then into his private office. He removed his hat and coat and hung them in a hidden closet behind a wall. The office was decorated with more oriental rugs and a large, polished mahogany desk, with two leather guest chairs in front and his own rotating leather chair behind. His chair sat in front of a wooden credenza that rested beneath a large panel of light boxes used for reading X-ray plates. The only whimsical bit of decor was the Phillies baseball hat that sat on the skull of his mounted skeleton. There were also a striped couch and a coffee table beneath the windows looking out on a view of the city. The window to the left of his desk presented a second urban view. His walls were filled with his many diplomas and award certificates and a large, framed copy of the Hippocratic Oath. Along the wall opposite the window was a floor-to-ceiling bookcase filled with his orthopedic reference books and his own bound writings. On the floor in front of the bookcase were large cardboard cartons stacked three high.

Outside his office door was a hallway connected to small rooms that consisted of his patient examination rooms and the utility rooms for patient medications and plaster cast applications At the end of the hallway were a room for taking patient X-rays and a room for the development and storage of the images. His patient assistant and X-ray technician inhabited this space.

His office manager and right-hand woman, Maria, entered his private office with his first cup of coffee of the day. Maria Cleopatra Gregorios was of Greek origin but was no Greek linguist, and she certainly did not understand Latin, so she was just as amused as the rest of the staff with Dr. Marks's morning greetings.

Maria was five feet four, slim, and had auburn hair (most of the time). Her prominent nose fit her face well. She said she was about the same age as Ham. She wore a starched white coat over her sweater and skirt. In fact, all of the women in the office wore either the long white coat over their street clothes or the nurse's outfit of a long, colorful shirt over pants. Ham, on the other hand, wore a suit and tie. He had had enough of starched white uniforms as an intern and resident.

Despite Maria's Greek heritage, Ham knew that she neither spoke nor understood Latin or Greek. But he got a kick out of the fact that her middle name was Cleopatra. It gave her a classical flavor.

"Those file boxes just arrived this morning, Doctor," Maria said while pointing to the large cardboard file boxes capable of containing thousands of pages of documents for the doctor's review.

"This cover letter came with the boxes from defense attorney Albert Broder," she continued as she handed a four-page, single-spaced letter to the doctor. "He made an appointment to talk to you about this case tomorrow morning. Is that all right with you?"

"That's fine. Thanks, Maria," Ham acknowledged.

Maria turned, her stiff white coat brushing against the office door, as she left Ham to read the letter and stare pensively at the large file boxes stacked against his bookcase.

The letter explained, in some detail, the medical malpractice case that Mr. Broder was defending and exactly what he would like Ham to do in his role as consultant forensic orthopedic surgeon. Mr. Broder had made it quite clear that this case was big. It involved suits against multiple people and organizations, potentially for millions of dollars.

There was even the possibility that a criminal charge of murder could be brought against the operating surgeon in the case, a circumstance that would involve a criminal defense attorney, beside Mr. Broder. It was a circumstance that Ham would have to consider in his evaluation of the medical facts of the case.

In brief, the case involved a suit brought by the wife of the deceased patient, in this case, himself a malpractice attorney, who had entered the University of Philadelphia hospital to undergo bilateral, total-hip replacements performed by the hospital's chief orthopedic surgeon. Forty-eight hours after the operative procedure, the patient died for unknown reasons.

The wife, representing the deceased lawyer's estate, was suing everybody: the surgeon, the hospital, the HMO that insured her husband, the anesthesiologist, the internist who cleared the patient for surgery, and the hospital consortium of which the hospital of the University of Philadelphia was just one part. Albert Broder, JD, was the lead defense attorney for all of the entities.

The plaintiff attorney, Claude Matthews, was the law partner of the deceased, Evan Stoner, Esq., in the law firm of Stoner & Matthews. He had also convinced the deceased's wife to initiate a criminal case for murder against the operating surgeon, Professor Edward Miller, MD, PhD, and FACS, since the doctor had previously lost a two-million-dollar medical malpractice lawsuit brought by Evan Stoner. To the plaintiff and her attorney, it was obvious that Stoner's death was the doctor's retribution. Why Stoner would want this man to operate on him in the first place was a curious question with an even more curious answer. In the first place, no other surgeon wanted to risk being sued by Stoner, and Dr. Miller with "evil and pathologically egotistical intent" convinced Mr. Stoner that he was the "most accomplished" and possibly "only" surgeon capable of doing this major surgery.

Stoner's wife, Marion, his *second*, was out for blood—blood from a Stoner. She would share any inheritance with Stoner's two children from his first wife. And besides, she was convinced, with the aid of her attorney, who was no devotee of Stoner and who himself had made a ninety-yard pass at Marion, that Stoner had cheated her in his prenuptial agreement by not listing all of his assets. It was a continuance of the fraud he had perpetrated during the divorce settlement with his first wife.

The widow was suing for damages for a number of reasons: lost earnings (the fifty-nine-year-old lawyer brought five to ten million dollars a year to the law firm and could be expected to continue to do so for many years), the pain and suffering Stoner endured, loss of consortium (a personal concept that reflected the normal sexual relationship between a man and his wife but was anything but normal in Stoner's case), loss to the children of a father's love and care (Ham laughed at that one), and the special medical costs of caring for Stoner in his last few days. Missing from this list was the actual causing of the death of Stoner, the punitive damage charges, and the charge of murder against the operating surgeon.

As it turned out, the filing of death charges was complex, requiring additional court maneuvering, and did not pay as well as loss of consortium charges anyway. The punitive damage request would require an additional legal filing. And the murder charge would be the job of the district attorney's office, if he could be convinced, and was actually just an attempt at leveraging the defense to come up with a whopping settlement. Marion did not actually care if Miller was charged and convicted. All she wanted was money. And some final revenge.

The reasons that Marion Stoner (through her lawyer) thought that she warranted all this money were many and varied. First in the list of complaints was that the double hip-replacement surgery was contraindicated because of preexisting medical conditions (which would be expanded upon later in the discovery process). Next, they claimed that Stoner was not properly informed that one of the possible complications of his surgery was death forty-eight hours after the operation. And they claimed the surgeon had not performed the surgery in a "workmanlike manner." In other words, he screwed up somewhere during the surgery. They further charged that there was improper pre- and postoperative testing, negligence in the postoperative care, and failure to obtain the proper postoperative consultants who could have prevented his death. Finally, they charged that the operating team had given the improper medication postoperatively.

Ham put down the letter and turned his attention to the three large file boxes. They contained, according to Broder's list, legal documents; depositions of various parties, including Marion Stoner, the two Stoner children, Stoner's first wife, operating surgeon Ed Miller, Stoner's pilot, Stoner's horse trainer (all of whom had visited him in the first forty-eight hours of his hospitalization), and the medical consultant who had cleared

Stoner for surgery; all of the hospital records; nurses' notes for the stay at the hospital, including the autopsy records; plus statements from investigators hired by the defense to dig into Stoner's life—and the lives of all the involved parties.

Ham's job was to determine "with reasonable medical certainty" that none of the people sued were responsible for Evan Stoner's death.

Ham thought, *Time to open Pandora's boxes!*

Chapter 2

Modus Operandi

The way of doing it

The hospital records that Ham perused first were voluminous. While some of the information was in computerized form, many records were still in longhand, the hand of a doctor or nurse. Nurses wrote clearly, but doctors, for some perverse reason, had abominable handwriting. Twenty billion federal dollars spent on electronic medical records couldn't correct any medical errors made by not being able to decipher a doctor's illegible scrawl. The pages had been scanned into a computer, but the handwriting often remained difficult, if not impossible, to read.

The preadmission history, physical examination, and presurgical medical consultation had cleared Evan Stoner for the bilateral, total-hip replacements necessitated by avascular necrosis. Avascular necrosis of the hip joints was a condition in which the bone cells of the ball of the hip died and the ball collapsed, leaving a deformed and very painful hip joint. The origin of the condition was known to be associated with diabetes mellitus (which Stoner didn't have), strange blood diseases (which he didn't have), deep-sea diving (which he didn't do), and alcoholism (which, it turned out, he had). However, 70 percent of the time no reason could be associated with the condition.

His liver function blood studies were abnormal, but other than that he passed his preadmission testing with flying colors.

Upon reaching the operating room, he was identified by his wristband, which listed his name, age, sex, and hospital file number. Also noted was the marked presurgical dressing on both hips, indicating that both were to be operated on—no possibility for a left-side or right-side mistake here. He had signed a standard hospital form that explained the upcoming procedures, including the anesthesia, the possible complications of the procedure (including death), and his alternatives. He could get up off of the gurney, if he so desired, and go home!

An intravenous line was established in his arm, and the board-certified anesthesiologist gave him a spinal anesthesia, which numbed him from the waist down. He would be awake during the operation but under medication that provided him with what the anesthesiologist called a "twilight sleep condition" as well as loss of memory of any of the sights or sounds that accompanied the procedure. This was the safest type of anesthesia for this patient.

The surgical team consisted of Dr. Miller, a resident orthopedic surgeon, a board-certified orthopedic surgeon serving as Dr. Miller's "hip fellow," and another orthopedic surgical resident. Surgical nurses were at the operating table and helping from the sidelines. The anesthesiologist stayed at the head of the table and tended to Stoner's comfort and vital signs.

The surgery proceeded with the usual cutting, tying of blood vessels, suturing, sawing, reaming, and placement of the plastic socket component and the metallic hip prosthesis without a hitch. Dr. Miller moved from one side to the other to perform the major portions of the surgery.

The anesthesia record noted a temporary drop in blood pressure when the metallic hip implants were hammered into place within the femoral shafts, but this quickly returned to normal. Two units of blood were given during the two-hour procedure, but they were autologous blood units that Stoner himself had given prior to surgery so there was no possibility of incompatibility. A postoperative X-ray showed the prosthetic implants to be in excellent position, and the patient was transferred to the recovery room.

After four hours of being monitored in the recovery room, Stoner was transferred to his private room while his intravenous line was still running. His postoperative orders included pain medication at first given intravenously, then intramuscularly, and finally by mouth. He was given several doses of antibiotics for twenty-four to forty-eight hours and was given low doses of heparin, a blood thinner, to prevent the formation of blood clots in his legs. Otherwise, clots might float in his bloodstream to his lungs as an embolism.

For the first day, he was allowed no visitors. But on the second day, not only was he allowed to see visitors but also he was allowed to sit on the side of his bed to converse with them for brief periods.

The nurses posted the visitor list. The list of people who visited him briefly on the second postoperative day included his wife, Marion; his two children; and his first wife's twin sister (who looked exactly like his first wife and had been, like his first wife, a nurse). The first wife did not appear. His personal pilot, his horse trainer, and finally the captain of his private yacht also visited him.

The nurse's notes recorded a perfectly benign postoperative course, according to the listing of vital signs and clinical notes.

After visiting hours, at approximately eight o'clock in the evening, the floor nurse entered his room to check on him. She found him unresponsive and not breathing. She immediately issued a code blue and within one minute the medical team was attempting to resuscitate Stoner.

At 8:10 p.m., the board-certified physician who headed the resuscitation team declared him dead, with the initial cause of death listed as "cardiac arrest" caused by probable "pulmonary embolism."

A nurse immediately notified his wife. She appeared with one of Stoner's children within an hour. After a tearful few minutes with Stoner, the dead body was moved to the hospital morgue to prepare for an autopsy, which was mandatory in the case of postoperative death.

Stoner was dead. Now Ham had to examine his life.

Chapter 3
Modus Vivendi

The way of living

Who was Evan Stoner? For Ham, the answer to this question came from the biographies, depositions, investigative reports, and expert opinion reports he dug out of the three large file boxes.

Evan Stoner was fifty-nine years old at the time of his death. He had grown up in Devon, Pennsylvania, the first son of a middle-class family living the mainline Philadelphia life. He attended Lafayette College and the University of Pennsylvania Law School. He was, for most of the time, a diligent, if not brilliant, student.

He married June Stewart, a working registered nurse, who helped support him while in law school (a reasonable bargain, according to the divorce settlement records). June had a twin sister, Susan, who married well by hooking up with a big pharmaceutical executive named Joseph Ralph. Ralph brought home a big salary and lots of executive perks, and Susan lived the high life for a time. Then lightning struck. Evan Stoner sued Ralph's company, Raven Drugs, over the side effects of one of its drugs and recovered a multimillion-dollar damage award. The financial loss essentially shut down the company, derailing the Ralphs' present and future ride on the high road.

June produced two sons with Evan and they were now twenty and twenty-three years old. They had barely spoken to their father in years. Stoner divorced June after ten years of marriage, and within a year he had married his beautiful, young, legal secretary, Marion Feld. Stoner and

Marion had no children. Marion had signed a prenuptial agreement, which left her very well off should Evan die or divorce her. Unfortunately for Marion, Stoner, allegedly in collusion with his partner, Clyde Matthews, had not listed all of Stoner's assets in the prenup. This essentially cheated Marion out of millions of dollars, should something unfortunate happen to their marriage—or to Stoner.

In life, Stoner was a tyrant. He was a tiger in court, ripping mercilessly through the flesh of his opponents. He started his own firm with his law-school classmate. Clyde Matthews was a brilliant but somewhat introverted man who stayed mainly in the background in the firm of Stoner & Matthews. Prior to joining up with Matthews, Stoner had worked for ten years in a law firm headed by an egomaniacal plaintiff attorney who had labeled himself "The King of Torts." Stoner swore he would dethrone "The King."

Stoner & Matthews took on malpractice and negligence cases against doctors, hospitals, HMOs, hospital associations, and pharmaceutical companies. And, as he told everyone, he "won them all!" Actually he won 60 percent of the time. Ham chuckled. *But who's counting?*

One of the suits was against Raven Drugs for an anti-stroke drug, Clearvasc, which had the unfortunate side effect of causing massive cerebral hemorrhages in patients who were sensitive to it. The drug had cost $500 million and had taken years of clinical trials to get to market. It had cost the company $5 million alone to defend the suit. Stoner won a whopping verdict of $1 billion—Ham exhaled while thinking, *That's nine zeros!*—after filing for punitive damages. The company filed an appeal but settled for $450 million. After paying expenses for experts, help from other attorneys, court and discovery costs, and the distribution of money to the plaintiff, Stoner's fee was $180 million. The case made him very rich but had occupied his time for four years, straining his relationships with his wife and family, coworkers, and colleagues.

It also hit close to home in another manner. His first wife's twin sister was married to Raven's vice president in charge of research. After the trial, Raven's stock dropped from eighty-five to ten dollars, placing the millions of stock options owned by Sam Ralph underwater, which reduced his net worth from $10 million to well under a million. This financial disaster caused a deep depression in the company vice president. He had to go on strong medication and never regained the company's respect.

Stoner had even previously sued his orthopedic surgeon, Dr. Edward Miller, for a total-hip replacement in which the operated leg was three quarters of an inch shorter than the normal leg. The doctor fought him long and hard, not allowing the insurance company to settle the case, stating that the patient's old, deformed hip socket was responsible for the shortening and not the surgery, which defense experts claimed was "superbly done." The case went to a jury trial, but just after the jury was picked the two sides settled for $2 million. Dr. Miller remained the Allister Macfarland Professor of Orthopedic Surgery and chairman of the orthopedic department of the University of Philadelphia hospital. He was an internationally renowned teacher and researcher with over two hundred publications to his name and was the author of two books on the surgery of the hip joint.

When he was asked at his deposition why he would undertake a difficult bilateral procedure on a patient who had sued him, Dr. Miller answered, "Even Mr. Stoner deserved the best when it came to surgical care." When queried by the plaintiff attorney as to whether or not he considered himself "the best surgeon" to perform the surgery on Stoner, Dr. Miller answered simply, "Yes."

Stoner's wife, on the other hand, when she was asked about the interview and examination before the surgery, said that Dr. Miller was "discourteous, brusque, and had an evil glint in his eyes." In hindsight, it seemed he considered the surgery an opportunity "to get back at Stoner." Stoner, his wife said, felt that Miller was the best surgeon in Philadelphia, and probably on the east coast, and that the suit years before was "just business" and "didn't cost him a dime."

Over the years, Stoner had become extremely wealthy. He had three homes, including a ten-thousand-square-foot manse with a pool, tennis court, and riding stables in Exton, Pennsylvania. The second was a large, modern Florida home on a golf course. It had a private airstrip for his twin-engine airplane. And his third was a brick-and-glass home on the beach in Loveladies, New Jersey.

Not only did he have his own plane and was himself a pilot, but also he employed a pilot who would bring his plane to him as needed. Or the Lear jet on which he shared time.

And horses. He had three in his stables in Exton for his wife to play with and two thoroughbreds that he kept under the watchful eye of a professional trainer at nearby Keystone Racetrack.

And, of course, he had a boat: an eighty-five-foot Hatteras motor yacht named *Retort*, which he kept at Harrah's Marina in Atlantic City. He employed a full-time captain and his wife as a mate.

He was mean, demanding, and egotistical. He had few true friends but plenty of buddies who he either made rich or used to become rich. And drinking buddies by the score: lawyers, insurance men and women, golfers, sailors, and equestrians. He drank alcohol for breakfast, lunch, dinner, teatime, and midnight snacks. His tolerance for alcohol was amazing. Instead of becoming drunken and outrageous, the more he drank, the more charming and disarming he became. As miserable as he was to other human beings when he was sober, he was a pleasure to be with when he was under the influence.

And women loved him. He was handsome, rich, and persuasive. His dalliances were legendary. And as long as no little Stoners appeared to make a claim on him, he could get away with it.

But, as usual—with the exception of Dorian Gray—this life of Stoner's took a considerable physical toll on him. His cholesterol and triglycerides were through the roof without medication. His GERD was just barely held in check with another prescription drug. Fine red veins were slowly but inexorably covering his nose, a visible sign of his alcoholism. But most of all, his liver was battered. Cirrhosis was the diagnosis. Enlarged, hardened, and vascularly compromised, the changes were stealthily advancing. Most metabolic bodily processes are controlled by the liver; so while Stoner's outward appearance changed very little, he was actually rotting away from inside.

Ham finished the pertinent records, and thought, *Whew, what a life! Now if I can only figure out what killed him.*

CHAPTER 4
CORPUS DELICTI

The dead body

The entrance to the university hospital was a pleasure to view. Gleaming marble covered the floor and walls, with the university emblem emblazoned ten feet high on the wall facing the entrance. However, this patient-pleasing facade completely disappeared beyond the steps down to the pathology department. Ham saw sterile, off-white walls and the names of subdepartments painted in black block letters on glass doors: "Hematology Lab," "Histology Lab," and "Pathology Department."

He opened the last door and approached a thirty-something brunette woman in a long white coat. "Dr. Marks to see Dr. Gross," he said.

"Oh, yes, Doctor. He's waiting for you in his private office. Go right in."

Ham opened the glass door marked "Peter Gross, MD, Chief of Pathology." The pungent odor of toluene and formalin straightened the hairs in his nose. It briefly took him back to his days spent dissecting a cadaver in medical school.

"Hi, Ham. Come on in and take a seat—if you can find one," Dr. Gross said, briefly looking up from his microscope.

Finding a seat was not as easy as it sounded. Everything—desk, seats, shelves, and even the floor—was covered with boxes of slides and department of pathology forms labeled with patients' names. Books and reprints from various pathological journals filled the blank spaces.

Ham moved a few boxes with their attached forms and sat in a wooden armchair with the Princeton University seal and motto, "Dei Sub Numine

Viget," which he knew meant "Under God's Name She Flourishes." Peter Gross was Ham's Princeton classmate.

"So you'd like to know what killed Evan Stoner, would you?" Gross said with a wry smile.

"Actually, I would," Ham said, moving his feet under his chair while trying to avoid crushing some glass slides in a pile on the floor near his chair leg.

"Well, let's look at the chart." Gross turned his attention from the slide he was viewing to a file filled with pages that were either copies from Stoner's inpatient chart or were compiled by the pathology department as it had investigated his death through laboratory studies, autopsy findings, and tissue samples.

The quick review of the data brought a frown to the pathologist's face, which was already creased by a multitude of wrinkle lines unretouched by Botox.

"Well, he wasn't in great shape, was he, Ham? His liver looked like an old leather boot that had been out in the rain too long—enlarged and cirrhotic. The booze was really killing this guy."

"Did it *really* kill him? I mean, did he die of liver failure?"

"Nooo. He still had a few years to go—but not much longer. All his liver functions were abnormal though, including his blood-clotting mechanism."

"Was that the key? His clotting mechanism? Did he hemorrhage?"

"Actually, no. He had considerable unclotted blood in his operative sites, and his hemoglobin had dropped from fourteen grams preoperatively to ten grams, despite being given two units of whole blood intraoperatively. But the nurses' notes don't describe a particularly wet dressing. But you already know that, don't you?" Dr. Gross knew Ham's propensity to memorize the pertinent clinical details of a case he was working on.

"Yes, he wasn't expected to need much in the way of prophylactic anticoagulation, except a bit of aspirin," Ham commented. "What about pulmonary or fat emboli?" Ham knew that his friend would get to this subject sooner or later, and he wanted it to be sooner.

One of the most common causes of sudden postoperative death, especially when the legs were the operative sites, was a pulmonary embolus. A blood clot could break off from a leg vein and pass through the heart and into the major blood vessels of the lungs. If the clot was large enough, it jammed the opening of one or more of the pulmonary blood vessels, causing a cascade of pulmonary and cardiac events that could lead to sudden death.

Fat embolism, on the other hand, took the same course but was derived from either fat globules mobilized from a fracture of a bone or reaming of the bone marrow in preparation for putting in a prosthesis, such as a total-hip replacement.

Ham knew that patients with poor liver function had difficulty handling the metabolism of fat in the bloodstream. In fact, the reason for Stoner's bilateral avascular necrosis of the hips was thought to be due to obstruction of the blood vessels in the femoral heads by fat globules.

"Well, that was originally thought to be the cause of death, you know," Gross stated. "And I did find both fat and microscopic marrow fragments in the pulmonary vasculature. But I didn't think it was enough to cause this man's death. I could be wrong, though."

But Gross had never been wrong in his clinical diagnoses in the many decades the two had known each other.

"Anything else of interest?" he asked.

"Well, he didn't die of a massive heart attack."

"Then what actually killed him?"

"His heart stopped beating," said Gross.

"That's a great help!" Ham said sarcastically. "Was that due to his operative procedure?"

"That sure didn't help—in a man with his liver status."

"Is there anything in the toxicology studies?" Ham persisted.

"No," said Gross while thumbing through the reports before him. "Certainly nothing that we routinely look for, such as amphetamines, alcohol, or barbiturates. He did have an elevated blood level of morphine, but he was on a postoperative morphine pump intravenously, so that's not unusual."

"Thanks a lot, Pete. I guess I'll see you at the next Princeton reunion, if not before."

"Okay, Ham. Good to see ya. Hope I was of some help to you." Gross turned his attention back to his microscope.

Ham gingerly rose and tiptoed among the slides until he reached the office door. He thanked the lady in the white coat and headed back to his office. He now had all the information that could be gathered from a corpus delicti.

CHAPTER 5

QUOD ERAT DEMONSTRANDUM

That which was evident

"Quod erat demonstrandum."

That was Ham Marks's greeting to Maria and his staff this a.m., as he walked through his office door. No one knew what that meant. Maria smiled. The rest of the staff just rolled their eyes.

"The defense attorney on that Stoner case—Mr. Sam Broder—is coming in to consult with you this morning, Doctor," Maria stated as Ham turned toward his private office.

"Okay, bring me some coffee, Maria, and let's get the show on the road."

"The coffee machine is broken, Doctor. I'll have to send out for some," Maria answered.

Maria would call The Little Greek's Restaurant. Maybe one of her relatives worked there, but they did deliver in a hurry, and their coffee was good. Corned beef special sandwiches as well.

At nine a.m., Sam Broder, Esq., from the law firm of Blank, White, and Broder, was ushered into Ham's consultation room. He carried two large briefcases, which he set down on the floor, and with a brief "Good morning, Doctor" started to unload the cases onto Ham's large desk.

"Sam, I already have a three-foot high stack of records to go through on this case," Ham quipped.

Sam Broder, a serious man who was seriously balding, and whose askew tie and unbuttoned white shirt showed that he was more serious about legal matters than he was about his dress, answered Ham with, "This guy, Bart Miles, wants to repaper our office walls with this case."

"Bart Miles? I thought Clyde Matthews was the plaintiff attorney!" Ham exclaimed.

"He is, but he turned the everyday battle over to one of his young attack dogs who wants to make a name for himself. Ham, we really need your help on this one!"

Broder was from a big defense firm of 150 lawyers. Ham had done work for this firm before.

"Well, Sam, I helped you on the defense of Dr. Stanley and you did just fine," Ham stated.

"Yes, we did get a defense verdict on that one, but all bets are off this time. We're talking *real* money here. They want nearly a billion dollars!"

"Wow!" Ham exclaimed as Sam Broder continued to pile deposition testimony after deposition testimony on his desk. "What's the chance of that happening?"

Sam Broder grunted but didn't answer at that moment. Ham took this time to muse on the state of malpractice in the Commonwealth of Pennsylvania as he waited for his coffee and watched Sam Broder set up for their meeting.

Statistics showed that 70 percent of malpractice cases ended in favor of the defense. This was once the case went to trial. The statistics didn't include the monetary settlements outside the courtroom. However, jury verdicts for the plaintiff, while only in the 30 percent range, had been moving, with alarming regularity, over the million-dollar mark.

Malpractice litigation is an expensive business, Ham thought. It created losses in time, effort, and money and caused psychological stress, particularly in doctors. Doctors certainly realized that they were human, and occasionally made mistakes, but almost all of them adhered to the Hippocratic dictum, "Primum non nocere." The first responsibility of the physician was not to harm the patient in an attempt to get him well.

Ham stepped around his desk and peered out the door of his office to see if Maria was coming with his coffee. He continued his musings.

Most defendant doctors were well trained and ethical. A mistake made by one of these doctors was not medical negligence; neither was a bad clinical result of treatment. Even the death of a patient was not necessarily due to malpractice. Medical negligence required a deviation from, or a failure to, adhere to accepted standards of medical practice (an intentionally vague concept).

The financial and psychological costs start when the patient first says, "Doc, I got a pain right here." The defense against potential claims starts with the ordering of more tests than are necessary, just to cover the bases. This "defensive medicine" is bad medicine.

Malpractice insurance premiums have certainly risen to obscene levels, Ham thought. Consequently, the strain on the medical system because of the lack of patient access to high-risk specialists—including obstetricians, general surgeons, vascular surgeons, cardiothoracic surgeons, orthopedic surgeons, and neurosurgeons—has become almost too much for the system to bear.

The legal eagles point to a study of questionable value by the Institute of Medicine, which found that between forty-four thousand and ninety-eight thousand annual patient deaths result from medical mistakes. "Clean up your act, or we'll clean it up for you," is the catchphrase of malpractice attorneys.

The medical insurance companies take shots from both sides. Lawyers claim that the companies are not run in a businesslike manner, with executives getting multimillion-dollar salaries plus perks. Doctors claim that the big companies have squandered their reserves on high-flying Internet stocks and are now taking their financial whipping out on hardworking physicians. The insurance companies deny everything, maintaining that they are run in the most businesslike fashion, and that their hardworking executives deserve their whopping salaries. What an unholy mess, Ham thought.

Ham returned to his desk and looked at Sam Broder, who was beginning to perspire and was mopping his brow with his crumpled breast-pocket handkerchief. *Lawyers have to eat too,* Ham reasoned, *and pursuing a malpractice case may cost them $100,000 or more, with expenses for various filings, expert witness fees, depositions, travel, and court costs. The defense bar is not a charity either; they are paid well by the insurance carrier or the self-insured entity (hospital, hospital system, or HMO).*

Punitive damages change everything. They are infrequently brought against a physician, since doctors don't usually have the net worth to warrant them and they are not covered by their insurance policies. But the big defendants could find themselves on the hook for hundreds of millions, or even billions, of dollars if they should be found by the jury to warrant the awarding of punitive damages for an act of medical negligence. So there was a clear and present necessity, in the Stoner case, for Ham's expertise to help the defendants, represented by Sam Broder, save potential truckloads of money.

Broder stopped mopping the beads of sweat from his brow, but there was visible fear on the face of this tough defense attorney. *Money and stress everywhere,* Ham thought, as he looked out his tenth-floor window onto a calm November day in the city of Philadelphia. The view was anything but awe inspiring, but there were better views elsewhere that reflect the power and money in the buildings and mini skyscrapers built since the overthrow of the "Billy Penn's Hat" building restriction in the last twenty-five years. Prior to that city regulation, no building was allowed to rise above the level of the hat on the statue of William Penn, the British founder of Pennsylvania, which rose above the dome of the city hall.

At that thought, Maria entered the office with his coffee. Ham returned to his desk, sat down, and started to read some of the documents laid out by Sam Broder.

CHAPTER 6
DEUS EX MACHINA

It came out of nowhere

Dr. Ruth Marks was a good-looking woman. She was five feet ten, had well-quaffed brunette hair and a beautiful face, and was in good physical condition from her tri-weekly workouts, as attested to by her toned arms and shapely calves. She stepped down with ease from her Mercedes SUV in the doctors' parking lot at the Bala Cynwyd Hospital.

She shut the driver's door and pointed her key at the lock for a remote closing maneuver. At that moment, she felt something like a pipe stuck into her back, just below her shoulder blades. She heard a low, growly voice say, "Dr. Marks?"

She tried to turn toward the voice, but the pipe in her back prevented her from doing so. She caught a glimpse of a man in a hooded sweatshirt standing just behind her with his arm outstretched and the pipe—or, for heaven's sake, a gun—pressed to her back. It was broad daylight and Dr. Marks, a pediatrician, could not believe that anyone would accost her in the doctors' parking lot.

"What do you want? I don't carry any drugs—or money."

"Get back in the car," the man growled.

"Why? What do you want?" Ruth asked, her face growing pale with a sweat starting, despite the cool November weather.

"Don't ask questions, or you might get hurt. Get back in the car!"

Ruth Marks unlocked her car door and stepped back into the driver's seat. The hooded man moved in front of the car, pointing a silver handgun at Dr. Marks through the windshield until he reached the passenger door. He jumped into the passenger seat, put on his seat belt, and pointed the gun at Ruth Marks. "Drive!" he said.

"Where?" Dr. Marks answered with obvious fear in her voice.

"Drive down Lancaster Avenue, and get on the Blue Route going south," the man said.

Dr. Marks did as she was told. She headed out of the parking lot, took a left on Lancaster Avenue, and drove to the entrance of the Blue Route going south. She entered the highway traffic. She did all this in silence, but once on the Blue Route she got up the courage to ask, "Where are we going? And why are you doing this?"

"Shut up!" the man said. "I'll tell you where we are going when we get there, and by the way, it's all your husband's fault."

"My husband?" Dr. Marks said. "What does he have to do with this?"

"If he hadn't stuck his nose into the Stoner case, you wouldn't be here now."

"Stoner case?" Dr. Marks said. "I don't know anything about a Stoner case."

"That's not the point. Your husband knows, and he should stop sticking his nose into something that doesn't have anything to with him."

Gathering some confidence, Dr. Marks said, "What do you have to do with the Stoner case?"

The man, who she could now make out as a swarthy fellow with a mustache and a goatee, said, "Never mind. I'm just the messenger. But if you don't want to get hurt, you'll tell your husband what happened today and convince him to pull out of the case."

At this point, the car had reached the entrance to I-95 going south. The carjacker said, "Turn here."

Dr. Marks entered the ramp to I-95 and proceeded south toward Wilmington, Delaware. Her mind was going a mile a minute. She figured that perhaps, if she didn't make any unnecessary moves or aggravate this man with a gun, she could get away without getting hurt.

As the car reached a roadside gas station and restaurant just off the highway outside Wilmington, the man said, "Turn off here, and get out of the car!"

She pulled the car into a parking spot, opened the door, and stepped out a bit shakily.

The man with the gun had undone his safety belt and jumped over the center console into the driver's seat. He grabbed the door handle and was about to shut the door when he looked at Dr. Marks and said, "And if your husband doesn't get out of the Stoner case, you'll lose more than your car the next time!"

With that, he slammed the door and drove off the ramp onto I-95.

Dr. Marks immediately reached into her pocketbook and pulled out her cell phone. The numbers blurred before her eyes and she had difficulty controlling her index finger while trying to punch in the numbers 911.

"Craaack, booom." Ham recognized the sound of his front office door closing as Sam Broder exited. At the same time, Maria appeared with a second steaming paper cup filled with hot coffee. It had a smiling Greek sailor on the face of the cup. Ham thanked Maria and took a very judicious sip of the coffee, knowing it was piping hot. He prepared to leave his private office for his examining rooms to see the first patients of the morning, but before he could reach the door his intercom buzzed. He returned to his desk and pressed "IC" on his phone console.

"Yes?" Ham answered over the speakerphone.

Maria's voice sounded high pitched and tremulous. "The Delaware State Police are on the phone, Dr Marks."

"Delaware State Police? What could they want?" Ham pressed the button to open the speaker on an outside line. "Hello. This is Dr. Marks. What can I do for you?'

"Excuse me, Dr. Marks. This is Officer Ralph Portino from the Delaware State Police."

"Yes, Officer Portino, what can I do for you?"

"Well, sir, do you have a wife named Dr. Ruth Marks?"

A bolt of fear went through Ham's body as he answered in a softer voice, "Yes. Why?"

"Well, sir, she's fine, but she's been carjacked. We picked her up on I-95 outside of Wilmington after she called 911. Would you like to speak with her?"

"Yes, please," Ham stammered.

"Ruth, Ruth, are you all right?" Ham yelled into the phone.

"Ham, I'm okay. Just a bit scared. This ugly man with a gun carjacked me from the hospital and told me to tell you to get out of the Stoner case. What's the Stoner case?" Ruth asked nervously.

Ham didn't know what to say. He was absolutely stunned by what he had just heard. "Don't worry about it, dear. The police are going to take you home, and I'll meet you there, okay?"

"Okay, Ham. Take it easy though. I'm all right, and I'll see you at home," Ruth said in as calm a voice as possible under the circumstances.

Ham grabbed his hat and coat, headed for the door to his office, and exclaimed to Maria, all in one swirl of motion, "Maria, I've got an emergency at home. Please reschedule my patients. I'll call you later!"

"Craaack, booom," the office door closed.

CHAPTER 7
CAVEAT EMPTOR

Let the buyer beware

Ham had convinced his wife to stay home from work while he worked on reviewing the Stoner matter, which he had explained to her in some detail. He told her that these unfortunate events that were happening to them were just attempts to intimidate him, but they really weren't dangerous (he hoped). Anyway, this is what he did for a living. She resisted, but finally agreed to do her research work from home and reschedule her patients for one week.

The paper cup with the little blue Greek sailor appeared on Ham's desk as he concentrated on the deluge of paper that represented legal material and medical material associated with the Stoner case. There were long depositions, taken under oath, from Stoner's surgeon, Dr. Miller; the orthopedic resident physician under Dr. Miller's supervision; the operating room nurse who assisted Dr. Miller; the resident during Stoner's double-hip replacement; the anesthesiologist; the nurses who cared for Stoner both in the surgical intensive care unit and on the hospital floor reserved for orthopedic postoperative patients; plus the three private-duty nurses assigned to take care of Stoner during the eight-hour shifts in each day. The depositions were filled with hundreds of pages of questions from lawyer Broder and answers from the deposed individuals.

In another brown cardboard box, Ham had another set of depositions to peruse from nonmedical individuals, including Stoner's wife (who was bringing the multiheaded malpractice suit), his first wife, his grown children, his first wife's twin sister, his pilot, his boat captain, his horse trainer—all people who had visited Stoner in the last forty-eight hours of his life.

In addition, of course, Ham had all the medical records contained in Stoner's medical chart: doctors' exams and consultations, nurses' notes detailing literally every minute of Stoner's postoperative care, plus all of the pre- and postoperative diagnostic studies (X-rays, blood studies) and his vital signs (blood pressure, pulse, respiration rate) for every hour of Stoner's hospital stay. Finally, he had the autopsy report that detailed each and every one of Stoner's postmortem organs. Plus toxicology reports from his stomach contents and blood were available to Ham.

While the enormity of the legal case, explained to him by Broder, rested in the back of his mind, Ham knew that his job, as it had been in the thousands of previous medico-legal cases, was to know every detail of these voluminous records by heart. It would require many hours of reading, analyzing, and memorizing but was a task that Ham's mind, which was able to retain millions of bits of information and organize them into some coherent theory, was certainly up to.

Since Ham knew that this particular case was going to require many hours of his most intense concentration, he had arranged his office schedule so that his patient care would begin in the afternoon, leaving him the whole morning to begin the task of processing the information concerning Evan Stoner and his death.

He absentmindedly reached for the steaming paper cup of coffee on the corner of his desk, and a flitting thought passed through his mind: *The office coffee maker must still be on the fritz.* It was nice of the office staff to order out for him—and he picked up the phone and dialed Maria's intercom number to thank her for the thoughtful deed. He certainly needed the caffeine kick before tackling the monumental task before him.

"Thanks for the coffee, Maria," he said. He always thanked his office staff for bringing coffee or lunch to his desk—in order to satisfy the pique that often accompanied the waitress-like duties that he often asked his staff to do for him, which they resented either by verbal or nonverbal signals.

"You're welcome, Dr. Marks, but I didn't bring you the coffee today," Maria answered in the typical hollow sound coming over an intercom.

"Well, I guess it was one of the other girls. Thank them for me. I certainly need the kick-start this morning. I'll be working on this mountain of records in the Stoner case. Give me a buzz when the first patient comes in."

"Okay, Doctor."

Ham lifted the steaming cardboard container, and as he cautiously brought the hot coffee to his lips he was mildly perplexed that the container had no lid on it. It was obviously brought to the office by The Little Greek's delivery person, and she always covered the coffee with a lid for transportation. She also supplied cream, sugar, and napkins, none of which appeared today. *Curious*, Ham thought as he viewed the coffee surface, which appeared to have the cream already added.

He took a careful sip of what he expected to be boiling hot liquid and was surprised to find the coffee lukewarm.

Disappointed at the temperature of his coffee, Ham set the container down on his desk and reached for Stoner's medical chart to start the review. As he placed the large file of documents on his desk, he tasted the bitter residue of his sip of coffee. *Needs more sugar,* Ham thought. He reached down to his lower desk drawer where he kept his stash of artificial sugar, salt, pepper, mustard, and ketchup for his at-the-desk lunches.

After picking up a packet of Sweet'N Low, Ham felt a kick all right. He felt as if he had been kicked in the head by one of Stoner's thoroughbreds! He thought for a moment that the top of his head was going to explode.

Just before he lost consciousness, he reached over to the intercom console and punched the "Page All" button. "Help me!" he croaked weakly. Then his body pitched forward, out of his chair and onto the floor.

"Whoa! What happened?" Ham sputtered.

He felt as though he had the hangover of the new millennium—and he didn't even drink! His head hurt, his vision was blurred, he had difficulty speaking, and his limbs felt like lead weights—too heavy to move.

He was on one of his examining room couches, IVs running in both of his arms. Big, burly EMTs were attending to his IV, monitoring his blood pressure, and unwrapping additional medications and syringes.

A policeman and Maria were standing at the door of the examining room. They slowly swam into his vision. "Where am I? What happened to me?" Ham asked again.

"It's all right, Doc. You're in your office and everything is under control," the EMT who was monitoring his blood pressure stated.

"Okay, that's good. Now will someone please tell me what happened to me."

"Well, we're not quite sure," the EMT said. "Maria here found you on the floor of your office and called 911. By the time we got here, you were unconscious and had a BP of three hundred over one seventy. We thought you had had a stroke. Maria here said you didn't have high blood pressure. Is that right, Doc?"

"Yes, that's right," Ham answered.

"So we gave you an IV sedative and your pressure's now down around one sixty over one hundred. What's it normally run, Doc?"

"About one thirty over eighty."

"Well, something gave it a real kick in the pants," the EMT joked.

"The only thing I had was a sip of coffee from The Little Greeks." Ham's mind was finally starting to clear.

"We'll take a sample of the coffee back to the lab for analysis," the policeman said. "In the meantime, Doc, you'd better go home and go to bed."

With that, the three EMTs and the policeman shifted Ham onto a gurney and whisked him out of the office and into a waiting elevator.

"Maria, call my wife—and cancel today's patients," Ham said, barely getting out the words before the elevator door closed.

Chapter 8
Odi et Amo

I hate, yet I love

Ham felt fine the next day. He drank tea. The personal attacks on him, related to the Stoner case, bothered him greatly. But he was not a quitter, so he decided to soldier on. The thousands of pages that he had reviewed began to form certain stories in his mind.

The Pilot

The Bloomingdale's bag and the gray captain's cap with its gold, glistening braid sat incongruously on opposite night tables in room 101 at the Motel 95 on route 95 between the Philadelphia airport and center city.

Two bodies—a man's and a woman's—lay next to each other on the rumpled bed. They were definitely alive, just exhausted and not from being up too late since daylight streamed through the partially closed window blinds. The man, who was muscular, tall, and slightly graying around the temples, moved his hand along the back and over the buttock of the prone woman. His fingers caressed her buttock lightly but missed the fine plastic surgery scars where her buttock joined her thigh. Scars that represented the reshaping she had had done a few years ago to "push back middle-age spread."

"Mmmmmm," the woman cooed as she turned her well-rounded body toward the man and smoothly moved on top of him as he rolled onto his back. She mounted him and started to move slowly and languorously. Her blonde hair and ample breasts (enlarged, unbeknown to the man, by the excess adipose tissue removed from her buttocks) hung down on to the man's chest.

"I could go on like this forever," she said as she sighed.

The man smiled, obviously enjoying himself, but remained silent. After a few more very sensual moments, he spoke softly. "I have to get back to the plane, darling. We're having an engine inspection at four."

She made a puckering motion with her mouth, as if to blow him a kiss, and moved off his body to sit on the side of the bed while holding his hand and looking at his face. "I suppose I'd better get home as well. Evan usually calls about four, and while the maid would tell him I'm out shopping if I wasn't there, I like to be home for his call."

The man got off the bed and started to gather his uniform and his underwear as he headed for the bathroom and the shower.

"Roger, dear, I have a really serious question for you."

"Yes, what's that?" the man answered, his hands full of his clothing.

"Well, come back here and sit on the bed," the naked woman said, beckoning with an index finger.

"Oh, no!" the man exclaimed. "You can't get me back in bed that easily. I have a job to do."

"I know, I know, but this has to do with your job."

"Okay," he said as he sat down on the bed with all his clothes on his lap. "What would you like to know about being a pilot?"

"Well, first of all, you control the plane, don't you?"

"Of course."

"So no matter what Evan did while he was on the plane, the plane was under your control, right?"

"Obviously."

"Soooo . . ." she cooed, "couldn't you pretend that the plane was in trouble, set it to go down with him aboard, and just jump off?"

The man was stunned into silence.

"What are you talking about? In the first place, there is always a copilot, so even if I went out of my mind or was incapacitated he or she would take over the controls. Second of all, the plane is flying at six hundred miles an hour. You can't just *jump off* a plane flying at six hundred miles an hour!"

"Oh, well," she said as she bent over to start to gather her own clothes. "It was just a thought!"

The Horse Trainer

Jeff Halloran slapped the rump of the magnificent stallion as he held on to the lead attached to a bit in its mouth. The large black horse quickly turned and showed its profile to the man standing next to the trainer.

"What a magnificent animal!" the man exclaimed. "Who does he belong to?"

"Well, the majority owner is Evan Stoner, the lawyer. Know him?"

"No, but I've heard of him. Pretty successful, right?"

"Yeah, right," the trainer said with obvious distain in his voice.

"Don't you train race horses for him?"

"Yes."

"Seems to me he almost had a Kentucky Derby winner one year. Were you his trainer?"

"Yes, but the horse wasn't his. I was training for another owner, and he threatened to fire me if I continued, so I never made it to the Derby."

"Whoa, that must have pissed you off."

"Yes, yes it did. But it was a long time ago."

Halloran reflected on those years. Years when his marriage broke up because Stoner and his wife were having an affair.

"Well, why do you continue to train for him? You're a well-known professional in your field now."

"I know," Halloran mused. "But he pays well."

Halloran wasn't going to tell this horse owner, who might use his services, that Stoner knew he was a reformed alcoholic and had threatened to "spread the word" if he ever dropped him. So Halloran would never train another horse in his lifetime. *Stoner's a son of a bitch!*

The Former Sister-in-Law

Susan Ralph looked exactly like someone else. That someone was her identical twin sister, Janet, who was Evan Stoner's first wife. But the two women were not alike except for their appearance. Janet, a former nurse

31

with two teenage children, was a long-suffering divorcee on a budget. It was a very nice budget, but as a single mother (Stoner had little to do with his children) she had to see to their education, maintain a roof over their heads, and put food in their mouths with the money Stoner had ultimately settled with her for—after a long and a bitter divorce battle. She was still, even after the settlement papers were signed and filed, investigating with her lawyer the high probability that Stoner had hidden certain assets from discovery during the divorce proceedings.

Susan had found herself a very rich scientist, Joseph Ralph, PhD, who had helped start a very profitable pharmaceutical company with a capital value of over a billion dollars at the time she married him. She had lived the high life sharing mansions, boats, travel, and expensive jewelry with her CEO husband. She had no children, and she liked that! But that was over a decade ago.

Now she made eggs and bacon for herself and her husband in her kitchen in her split-level home in a middle-class neighborhood. Her CEO husband was a psychological wreck. Even three or four of the newest and most powerful psychotropic antidepressive drugs could not lift him out of his severe depression. He needed hospitalization three or four times a year. The couple lived on his disability insurance and on the moderate investments that he had been able to accumulate before *it* happened. *It* was the malpractice suit Evan Stoner had brought against her husband's company, claiming that one of its premier drugs had brought about the death of his client. Stoner won that suit, and his client was awarded $1 billion in punitive damages (later reduced to $450 million). The loss of the suit and the bad publicity had destroyed the pharma company, bringing about bankruptcy. The financial ruin of the majority stockholders was rapid and dramatic. Her husband lost tens of millions of dollars. His millions of stock options were worthless, and his pension plan and golden parachute agreement, which would have entitled him to several million dollars a year after his retirement, disappeared completely.

Dr. Ralph suffered a complete mental breakdown and had never fully recovered.

"Would you like some more eggs, dear?" she asked her husband who was sitting at the breakfast table, his head hung down in an obviously despondent posture.

"*Uhmmmmm,* I guess so," he barely answered.

That son of a bitch Stoner should die—slowly—for this, she thought.

The three people whose rationale for doing in Evan Stoner had all been visitors to his hospital room postoperatively. In addition, his former wife, a nurse, and her two children, all of whom Stoner had treated like dirt, had visited and had also been deposed.

Wow, thought Ham. *What a list of characters who all had a reason to at least cheer at his death, if not benefit from it.* His present wife, who was bringing the suit for his estate, would benefit the most, assuming there wasn't some restrictive prenuptial agreement. He would have to check that out with Broder.

CHAPTER 9

RES IPSE LOQUITOR

It speaks for itself

At the end of his workday, Ham closed the heavy doors of his office building and stepped into the cold November wind. It was raining, and he bent his head to allow his hat brim to protect his face from the beating drops of water.

After few steps, he made a quick right-hand turn onto Rittener Street and headed for his parking garage. The stark light from the sodium vapor lamps gave him the visage of a giant hulk moving through the night. He had gained a few pounds, and perhaps lost the best part of an inch in height from his days as a heavyweight wrestler for Princeton. But at six feet three and 230 pounds, he was an impressive figure nonetheless. Perhaps a bit slower than in his undergraduate days, but he could still move about the squash court well enough to beat most opponents. And heaven help them if they crashed into him running for the ball.

He passed by the doors of the DAR Club and the print shop. Both were closed, their doors locked and their lights out. As he passed a dark alley, wet falling leaves blew past him and landed on the slick cement. He made a mental note to watch his step, as he surveyed his surroundings, and he adjusted the briefcase in his hand so that it acted as a balance to his weight. He was particularly aware of his footing as he approached the shiny metal surfaces over cellar openings and over access boxes to Procast cable TV underground lines.

He began to think about the day's activities. Just as his mind got in gear, he heard a low, muffled voice from behind him. "Hold it, Doc!"

Ham was used to panhandlers on the street, but he knew to ignore them and keep on moving. But this one called him "Doc," and that was just enough to get his attention. He partially turned around and saw, silhouetted in the streetlamp's light, a slim figure wearing a baseball cap backward and holding what looked like a baseball bat in his hand. The figure remained silent but brought the baseball bat into an upright position and began to tap it on his opposite hand.

Ham began to turn away, but as he did he noted movement out of the corner of his eye as the figure approached him with the baseball bat raised above his head. Reflexively, Ham swung his briefcase to ward off the baseball bat. At the same time, utilizing some long-forgotten instinct, he swept his left foot out and behind the right foot of his attacker in an attempt to knock him off his feet.

At that moment, fortune stepped in. The attacker's right foot slipped on wet leaves, leaving him without a leg to stand on after Ham's leg whip, and he fell flat on his back, exposing a metal plate with the shiny letters "PROC—."

Ham fought back the instinct to fall on the figure and pin him to the ground in a wrestling mode. Instead, he dropped onto one knee, but that knee was on the chest of the supine figure. His 230-pound body held the 160-pound man immobile. Ham quickly disarmed his attacker and, resting the aluminum bat on his throat, said, "What is your problem?"

"No problem, no problem, Doc!" the slim figure shouted in a much higher-pitched voice than he had previously used to call for Ham's attention. "Let me go, and I'm outta here!"

Ham could now see the thin, swarthy face of the man before him. "Do I know you? How do you know I'm a doctor?" Ham blurted out.

"She told me. She described you!"

"Who did? Who sent you here to hurt me?"

"I don't know, honest, Doc! She called me on the phone and said she'd pay me five hundred dollars to beat you up and give you a message."

"What's the message?"

"Forget Stoner!" the supine man blurted out.

"What's that mean?" Ham asked the man who was now shaking beneath his weight.

"I don't know, man. That was the message I was supposed to give you."

"What's your name?" Ham continued.

"Hit man! They call me hit man!"

"Okay, hit man, but let's see what your momma calls you," Ham said as he reached into the back pocket of the immobilized man and extracted his wallet.

"Amos Bardon, age eighteen, 2675 Wharton Street," Ham read as he removed the man's driver's license and threw the wallet into his face.

"Okay, Amos, I got the message. Now you get the hell outta here before I whack you in the head," Ham stated menacingly as he grabbed the bat and stood up, taking his weight off of the younger man's body.

Amos quickly recovered his upright posture and ran down the street, disappearing into the darkness.

Ham started to shake at the realization of the threat to bodily harm that he had just avoided—plus the exertion of this unexpected—even by himself—physical response.

He walked on down the street, with his briefcase in one hand, and the aluminum bat in the other.

"Is it your turn at bat, Doc?" the garage attendant quipped.

"Nope, Lester. I think I just hit a home run!" Ham answered as he got into his car, gave the attendant a two-dollar tip, and drove home.

His thoughts, as he maneuvered through the narrow streets of Philadelphia toward the Schuylkill Expressway, focused on whom he should tell first about this latest encounter with evil. Should he call the Philadelphia Police? Should he talk to his wife? That might just scare the hell out of her! Maybe he should just keep the whole story quiet but bring it up with Linda Carter, an FBI agent he was scheduled to meet with in his office in a few days to discuss his wife's carjacking.

CHAPTER 10
ALIA JACTA EST

The die is cast

Ham strolled down the polished linoleum halls of the university hospital. He had just visited a patient for a consultation. He rarely hospitalized a patient of his own these days, since he had given up operating. But he often saw patients from some of his old referring physicians for nonoperative orthopedic problems that arose while the patients were inpatients for surgical or medical problems. The patient he had just visited had developed severe sciatica while hospitalized on the surgical service for a cancer operation. Ham had examined her and written orders for certain pain-relieving modalities (medication, physical therapy, and proper manipulation of the bed controls to flex the patient's knees and trunk to relieve any stretch of the sciatic nerve). He also had ordered a number of diagnostic tests to rule out the possibility that the patient was suffering from metastatic disease of the spine as a cause of the back and leg pain.

Even though he no longer spent time in the operating room, he still roamed the hospital floors frequently as he taught medical students, interns, and residents—often at the bedside. So he was still a familiar fixture in the hospital.

He waved to a few familiar faces among the nurses and doctors on the floor as he headed for the elevator, which would take him to the lobby. As he rounded the corner to the elevator waiting area, he heard the familiar *ding* of an arriving car, and he thought, *Must be my lucky day!* He was about to enter the elevator as the doors opened, but an orderly was pushing out a patient on a gurney and he had to step back to let them pass.

He stepped back into the elevator car and pushed the button for the lobby floor. As he did, a strange feeling passed over him, as if, as they say, someone had just walked over his grave. Something had just happened to him—but what was it? Something about the orderly aroused some sort of memory. He had never seen the man before, but that wasn't unusual. Orderlies, as opposed to nurses and doctors, came and went. Other than a few operating room orderlies, whom he recalled seeing on numerous occasions as they helped him move his patients on and off the operating table, he couldn't remember the name or face of a single orderly in the hospital in over thirty years of being on the staff. They were virtually invisible but always present.

So what could have been so special about this particular orderly? Ham tried to reconstruct in his mind just what the orderly had looked like. He recalled, *Dark*. He remembered, *Thin*. He probed his own mind and thought, *Mean looking with a goatee*. Now where had he seen someone like that? Then it hit him with a feeling of fear and loathing! He had never seen the orderly before, but his wife had described the man to a T. He was the man who had carjacked her, and threatened to do worse if Ham didn't give up his investigation in the Evan Stoner case!

Ham immediately changed direction and headed toward the hospital security office. The officer at the desk was reading some notice when Ham interrupted his concentration with, "Excuse me."

"Yes, sir, what can I do for you?" the uniformed officer immediately responded.

"I'm Dr. Marks—orthopedic service."

"Yes, sir, Dr. Marks. What seems to be the problem?" the officer asked with apparent interest.

"I just saw an orderly leaving the orthopedic floor with a patient. I want to ask him a question, but I don't know his name or how to locate him. Could you help me?"

"I'll certainly try, Doc, but we have a hundred orderlies here at the university hospital, and they are always coming and going. Not a very stable job position. Low pay, not great hours. Most of them are foreigners who apply for temporary work. Can you describe him? We do have photos of each orderly in the computer for the identification tags they must wear. Maybe we can match your description with your man's picture."

"That would be great," Ham said as he sat in the wooden armchair in front of the security man's desk. The officer turned his computer screen slightly so that both he and Ham could view it simultaneously.

"Let's see," Ham began. "He was dark skinned but not African American. *Swarthy*, I would call him. He had a small mustache and a goatee."

"That should give us enough to get a start on his identification," the security officer stated as he punched a number of keys on his computer keyboard. "I have six men who have mustaches and goatees. Take a look." The guard turned the screen toward Ham, and Ham studied the six photos.

The choice wasn't difficult. "That's him." Ham indicated by placing his index finger on one of the photos.

"Okay, let's see who that is," the guard stated as he punched a few more keys. "Here he is. Mohammed El Said, from Saudi Arabia originally. Been in this country for three years. Has the proper credentials, even worked as an orderly at Johns Hopkins in Baltimore, and his references checked out. Been here for about a month. Got no complaints filed against him. What's your problem with Mr. El Said, Doc?"

"No problem, I'd just like to ask him a question about a patient," Ham lied. He quickly wrote the essential information from the computer screen into the small notebook he always carried in his breast pocket. El Said was five feet ten, 155 pounds, and thirty-six years old. Unless he had a gun, which was most unlikely, he shouldn't present much of a threat when and if Ham had the opportunity to confront him.

"Where can I find him?" Ham asked as he put his notebook away.

"Well, Doc, the orderlies sit around in a vending room—you know, coffee and doughnuts—down in the subbasement waiting for work calls. It's room SB16. You want me to give them a ring and see if Mohammed is there?"

"No thanks, Officer. I'll stop down there. I don't want to disrupt his work schedule by having him wait for me. Thanks for your help." Ham rose from the wooden desk chair and offered his hand to the guard.

"No problem, Doc. That's what we're here for," the officer said with a smile as he shook Ham's hand.

Ham left the security office and took the elevator down to SB. As the elevator doors closed behind him, he found himself in a dimly lit hall with gurneys and other mobile equipment stacked against the light-green walls. *God, I hate that color! Why on earth would anyone paint any structure, except perhaps a prison, that nauseating color? It must be something psychological.*

39

Ham began his search for the vending room where he expected to find Mr. El Said. He heard voices ahead, and soon saw a lighted door in front and to the left, down the long hall. He approached the door and immediately observed some five or six men, in white uniforms, chatting and drinking coffee. *Women never become orderlies,* he thought. *It certainly can't be that the job is too hard. Women become soldiers, police, and fire persons—another interesting enigma,* he thought as he entered the well-lit room and the conversations ceased.

"Yes, sir. What can we do for you?" one of the orderlies who was facing the door asked politely.

"I'm looking for Mr. El Said," Ham answered. "Is he here?"

"No," the polite orderly answered, "but he told us he would be in room 103 if anyone asked for him."

"Fine. I'll look for him there," Ham said as he turned to leave the vending room.

"Who should I tell him is looking for him? If you can't find him, I mean," the orderly asked reasonably.

"Just a doctor who wants to ask him about a patient he recently moved," Ham lied.

Ham moved back into the dimly lit corridor and started looking for a door with "103" on it. He followed the numbers down from 110 and finally came to a closed wooden door with the inscription "103, Equipment" painted on it—unbelievably in the same nauseating green color that covered the walls. *Definitely a coordinated effect,* Ham thought wryly as he approached the door and knocked.

"Hello, Mr. El Said!"

No response.

"Hello, anybody in there?" he tried again. After a short period of silence, Ham tried the doorknob and found it unlocked. He entered a well-lit space, about six feet wide, whose depth he couldn't determine because of the shelves and cleaning equipment that obscured the back of the space.

The room smelled so strongly of disinfectant that Ham sneezed from the nasal irritation before he could call out. "Mr. El Said, are you back there?"

No sooner had Ham stepped fully into the foul-smelling equipment room than the wooden door closed behind him with a muffled *click.*

Must be on a spring closure, Ham thought, although he couldn't recall pulling against a spring when he opened the door.

Ham's thought processes were suddenly short-circuited when, right after the door closed, the lights went out.

"Hey, what's going on?" he cried as he turned to find the door handle in the dark.

Finding the doorknob wasn't much of a problem, but it was locked—from the outside!

"Hey, anybody out there! Open the door!" Ham bellowed as he pounded on the thick, wooden door. He stopped momentarily to listen if there was any response from the outside. There wasn't. As he pounded with his fist on the door, in the dark, he noted a change in the aspect of the darkness. Confused, he stepped away from the door and quickly noticed that someone on the outside was closing off the slit of light coming from underneath the door!

"Hey, cut it out! Let me out of here!" he protested. His mind whirled in confusion and then cleared itself like an opening computer screen. Not only was he in a locked room in the pitch dark, but also the only supply of air had just been closed off! The overwhelming smell of the place became even more pronounced. And Ham realized with an involuntary shudder that if he didn't get out of this room quickly, he would be overwhelmed by the toxic odor and lose consciousness.

He tried to break the door down, first with his shoulder—suffering a painful blow. Then he tried to kick the door, but without any leverage his kick was totally ineffective.

Okay, Ham, it's think or die. Panic will kill you. No light! The switch must be on the outside. No phone! I don't even have my cell phone. The damn thing is still in my car! Think man, think! Fire alarm! There must be a sprinkler head in here—particularly with all this volatile cleaning material. But it's pitch dark, I don't know where the sprinkler head is, and I can't reach it anyway! Reach!

He recalled the mops and broom sitting around the room that he had noted before the lights went out. He reached out with both arms and began a sweep in the dark. Suddenly his hand touched a mop or broom handle and he grabbed on to it like a drowning man. Swinging it up to the ceiling, he found that it easily reached to the ceiling. *Thank God!*

He immediately began sweeping the ceiling, feeling for an obstruction that hopefully would be a sprinkler head. Suddenly the broom struck something. Stopping his sweeping motion to get his orientation to the obstruction in the dark, Ham held the broom handle in place while he moved directly under the obstruction. As he stood in place, looking up at the darkened ceiling, he began to feel faint. He didn't have long before he lost consciousness, and lost any chance of getting out of this death trap.

Quickly, Ham began to strike the object on the ceiling. He missed several times, but finally he gave it a mighty swat and the obstruction gave way. Suddenly water poured down on him, soaking him instantly. That wasn't good! But at the same time, Ham heard the fire alarms go off all over the floor. Hoping that security could identify the alarm that he had activated and quickly come to his rescue, Ham huddled into a corner of the closet, trying to avoid the worst of the deluge.

He soon heard loud voices outside the locked door, and within minutes someone unlocked and opened the door to room 103.

Ham stumbled out into the light and into the arms of the security guard who had helped him locate El Said.

"Doc, Doc! What were you doing in there?" the guard queried.

A disoriented and soaked to the bone Ham mumbled, "You told me to come here. I was looking for Mohammed El Said, and someone locked me in."

"Jeez, Doc, I'm glad we found you so quickly. The smell of that cleaning stuff in there can kill you."

"You're telling me," Ham answered with a shiver as someone threw a blanket over his shoulders and helped him to the elevator.

CHAPTER 11

HUSTERON PROTERON

The last is first

Ham recovered from his closet episode over the weekend, prescribing lots of sleep and chamomile tea with honey for himself. He was in his office early Monday morning to review more depositions taken in the Stoner case.

"The FBI agent is here to talk to you about your wife's carjacking," Maria said as she appeared at his door. She was filled with disbelief that this visitor should be the first to see her boss in his orthopedic surgical office this morning.

"Okay, Maria, send him in."

"It's not a him, Dr. Marks," Maria remarked.

"Oh that's right, Maria, send her in then."

Maria disappeared from the office doorframe.

She reappeared within a minute. "Dr. Marks, this is Agent Carter to see you."

Maria stepped aside, and in walked Agent Linda Carter. She was blonde, blue-eyed, five feet six, trim, and dressed in a navy suit jacket and skirt with white piping on the jacket.

She extended her hand to shake Ham's. "Good to meet you, Dr. Marks. Or maybe not so good," she said as she grasped Ham's big hand and gave it an almost masculine squeeze.

"My pleasure entirely, Agent Carter," said Ham with obvious sincerity.

"Call me Linda, please," she said as she presented Ham with her badge and credentials. Ham examined her FBI identification badge and said gallantly, "Your picture doesn't do you justice, Linda."

"Those ID pictures never do, Dr. Marks."

"And you can call me Ham."

"Well, thanks, Ham. And now let's figure out what exactly is happening to you and your family," Linda stated matter-of-factly.

"Please sit down, Linda. But before you do, please answer an old scientist's curiosity."

"Sure, Ham, shoot!"

"Exactly!" said Ham brightly. "Where on earth, in that great-looking outfit you're wearing, do you hide your weapon? I assume you do have a gun somewhere."

Linda laughed, and with one swift motion reached behind and under her tight-fitting jacket and presented Ham with a gray Beretta pistol.

"There you are, Ham. But remember curiosity got the cat killed," Linda said with a smile as she replaced her weapon and sat in the upholstered chair in front of Ham's desk.

"Now, why don't you start at the beginning and tell me what's going on. All I've been told is that some 'foreign-looking guy' carjacked your wife over the state line into Delaware, demanding that you stop some investigation or worse things would happen. Is that the straight story?" Linda asked in a businesslike fashion.

"Well, it's a bit more complicated than that. Do you want to take notes?" Ham asked.

"Don't worry about that, Ham. I'm a pretty good listener. I'll write up my report after our interview. I don't like to break up our conversation with note taking."

Ham was impressed.

"Interesting. I do the same when I'm trying to figure out what occurred in an orthopedic case. Where did you go to undergraduate school?" Ham asked, thinking that perhaps he had a young Princeton graduate to deal with.

"I went to Yale. And then did graduate work in criminology at Harvard," Linda responded.

"Well, we have Harvard in common, Linda, but I graduated from Princeton—a long time ago."

"I know. Class of '67, right?"

"Right, Linda. I guess you Yalies do your homework."

"You bet, Ham. Now let's get back to the story at hand," Linda said, trying to redirect the conversation back to the case and away from Ivy League competition.

"Why don't you start from the beginning?" Linda directed.

"Fine," Ham said as he spun in his big desk chair and pointed to the piles of documents and depositions sitting on his credenza. "I guess it all starts here, with the Evan Stoner case."

"Tell me about the case," Linda directed.

Ham spent the greater part of the next hour giving Linda all the details of the case that started with the death of Evan Stoner, Esq., malpractice lawyer, after bilateral, total-hip replacements at the University of Philadelphia hospital. Ham presented the FBI agent with all he knew so far about the case. He filled in the details he had gleaned from defense attorney Broder about how Stoner's second wife, Marion, was pursuing the case through Stoner's former law partner, Claude Matthews, and how the lawyer was considering punitive damages in the millions, as well as a murder charge against the surgeon. Ham then moved to the details of the case history, including the surgery, the postoperative care, the known details of Stoner's death, and the inconclusive autopsy report.

Finally, Ham recited the stories he had learned from attorney Broder and the depositions he had so far reviewed about the visitors Stoner had to his hospital room postoperatively. Those included his wife, a victim of Stoner's philandering who was having an affair with the lawyer's personal pilot; Stoner's first wife, whose children allegedly had been cheated by the fallacious divorce agreement Stoner forced upon her; the first wife's twin sister, a nurse whose husband had been almost bankrupted by Stoner's suit against the pharmaceutical company where he had been an executive and held millions of dollars worth of stock and options that were now almost worthless.

The final two players who were entitled to hold a grudge against Stoner were his horse trainer, Al Finney; and the surgeon Miller. Finney had been cheated out of a training job with a potential Derby winner by Stoner's threat of spreading a rumor of alcohol abuse to other horse owners, and Finney suspected Stoner of having an affair with his wife. Miller was a proud surgeon stung by the two-million-dollar verdict won by Stoner against him in the past.

Ham took a deep breath and was about to continue his tale with the details of the multiple attempts someone had organized to keep him from investigating Stoner's death, when the intercom on his desk buzzed.

"Excuse me for a moment, Linda, while I answer this. It must be important since Maria knows you're here and I don't want to be interrupted."

"No problem, Ham. You go right ahead. If you want me to leave the room, I'll be happy to do that," Linda offered.

"No, you sit right where you are," Ham responded as he pressed the intercom button.

"Dr. Marks, someone from the American Academy of Orthopaedic Surgeons in Chicago is on the phone and insists on speaking with you," Maria said.

"Thanks, Maria. I'll take the call," Ham said as he pressed the button on his phone to turn off the intercom. He was poised to open the blinking phone line and said, "Linda, stand by. I don't know what this is all about, but the AAOS is the organization that gave me my orthopedic board certification thirty years ago."

Ham punched the line button on his phone console. "Hello, this is Dr. Marks."

"Dr. Marks, this is Stacey Malloy. I'm the assistant to the executive director of the American Association of Orthopaedic Surgeons, Dr. Marvin Alexander."

"Yes, Stacey, what can I do for you?"

"Well, Dr. Marks, I'm sorry to have to inform you that a complaint has been filed against you with the ethics committee, which requires a response from you, in person, here in Chicago."

"A complaint? What kind of complaint?"

"I can't tell you much about it, Doctor, other than it pertains to false orthopedic opinions you have provided in a malpractice case involving a surgeon at the University of Philadelphia, a Dr. Miller."

"Stacey," Ham responded incredulously, "I've been asked to provide an opinion in defense of Dr. Miller, not against him. And, incidentally, I haven't provided any opinion yet, either in writing or by deposition. So how can anyone file a complaint against me in this matter?"

"I don't know, Doctor. As you no doubt know, this is a new procedure, just introduced by the association in order to prevent false orthopedic testimony being presented by association members who present themselves as experts in malpractice cases. Anyone who is affected by the testimony that they consider false and below the standards of the association may file a complaint. And our bylaws clearly indicate that the association member against whom such a complaint is lodged must appear within ten days of notice before the ethics committee or risk having his or her board certification revoked.

"Would you like to schedule your appearance now, or would you like to call me back later today with a date for your appearance?"

"Stacey, I think I'll take the second choice and call you back," Ham answered, realizing that he wasn't going to get anywhere arguing the illogicality of this ethics complaint with this lady. She was just doing her job.

"All right, Dr Marks. I'll be waiting for your call. Good-bye."

"Good-bye, Stacey," Ham said as he clicked off the phone line button and sat back in his chair, staring at Linda with a puzzled look.

CHAPTER 12

POST HOC, ERGO PROPTER HOC

One thing causes another

Ham was drinking tea at his desk. Tea had become his drink of choice since the episode with his laced coffee. He drank it in a glass. It was clear—no milk or cream allowed. He inspected his tea bag very carefully before use. A well-attached tag was a necessity.

The hot water was supplied only by Maria. *It's not that I don't trust the Greeks, but forewarned is . . . And once burned . . . And all that stuff.*

It turned out, according to the Philadelphia Police Laboratory, that his *killer coffee* had been adulterated with pseudoepinephrine, or Sudafed, a drug found in cold and cough medicine. How it had gotten into his coffee—or how the hell the coffee cup had gotten onto his desk—he had no idea.

In fact, as he sat there surrounded by the thousands of pages of facts about the life and death of Evan Stoner, he had no idea why the potentially deadly events of the past few days had occurred to him and his perfectly innocent wife.

He had been threatened before in his medico-legal practice, but with legal action—malpractice suits or threats of perjury charges. Never with physical harm.

He tried to tie all the events together to determine who could possibly be responsible for them.

All of the actions—his wife's carjacking, the *killer coffee,* the hit man's appearance, the closet job, and the AAOS censure—involved the Stoner case. But how would anyone even know that he was involved in the case? Only Sam Broder and his staff, and his own office staff, had any inkling of his participation.

It was early days. He hadn't written anything about Stoner to anyone yet. Maybe the plaintiff, Mrs. Stoner, and her lawyer knew he had been asked to consult in the case, but there really was no need for them to know that he was involved until he had issued some written opinion. What if he had turned down the assignment?

And why such dastardly actions? Stoner was a malpractice lawyer, for heaven's sake—not a Mafia hit man! At least Ham didn't think he was a Mafia hit man!

What else could connect the characters involved—an adolescent thug, a malevolent Saudi hospital orderly, and the American Academy of Orthopaedic Surgeons?

The hit man had said that a woman had contacted him and told him to "beat up" Ham. *What woman?*

Then Ham had a thought. He turned to his desk telephone and punched Maria's intercom number.

"Yes, Dr. Marks?"

"Maria, would you please get the American Academy of Orthopaedic Surgeons office in Chicago on the phone for me."

"Of course, Dr. Marks."

Within a minute, Ham's phone buzzed. Ham picked up the receiver and said, "Hello."

"The American Academy of Orthopaedic Surgeons. How may I direct your call?"

"Could I speak with Stacey Malloy, please? This is Dr. Ham Marks from Philadelphia."

"Of course, Dr. Marks. One moment please."

Ham sat back in his chair.

"Hello, this is Stacey Malloy."

"Ms. Malloy, this is Dr. Ham Marks in Philadelphia. You called me a few days ago about a complaint that had been registered against me for my testimony against Dr. Miller in the Evan Stoner matter. Do you remember?"

"Of course, Dr. Marks. Have you decided on a date that you would like to appear before our Grievance Board?"

"No, not yet, Stacey, but I did want to get more information from you about the complaint. You recall that I told you that I was asked to give an opinion on behalf of Dr. Miller, rather than against his action, and that I hadn't written anything yet. So there was no way for a complainant to know what my opinion was. As a matter of fact, even *I* don't know what my opinion will be."

"Yes, Dr. Marks. I remember your comment to that effect, and I wrote your comments into the computer log on the case. But I told you that I don't handle the details of these actions. I just arrange to have the accused doctors appear before our board here in Chicago."

"Does your computer log tell you who lodged the complaint, Stacey?"

"It does, but I'm not allowed to give that information out over the phone. Once I arrange for your appearance, you will get a package from the academy, naming the complainant and stating the complaint, as it was received by us."

Ham hesitated for a moment.

"Ms. Malloy, can you at least tell me whether the complaint was called in by a man or a woman?"

"Well, I guess that wouldn't hurt. It was called in by a woman. The written complaint was to follow within forty-eight hours—but I notice that no written response has been received by this office as yet."

"Thank you for that. Could I ask you for one more favor?"

"What's that, Dr. Marks?"

"When you receive that written complaint, would you please call me again and then I'll give you a definite date for my appearance."

"Certainly. I'll mark that on the computer log and I'll be happy to follow through with a call to you when we receive the written complaint."

"Thank you, Stacey."

"Thank you, Dr. Marks."

Ham hung up the phone. He had a feeling that he would never hear from Ms. Malloy again.

But at least he had learned that a woman had called the academy, just as a woman had tasked the hit man. But what woman, and how was she involved in the Stoner matter?

At that moment, his intercom buzzed again. Ham punched the blinking light.

"Dr. Marks, you have a call on line one from Agent Carter."

"Thanks, Maria," Ham said as he punched the button to open line one. "Linda, what can I do for the FBI today?"

"Ham, I have some information that may be of some interest to you."

"What's that?"

"The FBI office in Washington, DC, has received some chatter from NSA concerning your friend Stoner and a friend of his, a Saudi sheikh who runs an Arabian stud farm in Kentucky. It's just chatter, but it certainly appears to relate to your case."

"Yes, it sounds like it does. NSA, huh? Them's big initials, Linda—maybe bigger than FBI, at least involving more of a *foreign* connection." Ham almost said "terrorist connection," but even he appreciated the *big ears* that were out there listening.

"Yes, I thought so too," Linda said circumspectly. "I'm thinking of visiting the sheikh in Kentucky. Would you like to come along, since you started all this?"

"I sure would," said Ham, thinking about a diversion from Philadelphia in November.

"I'll pick you up at nine tomorrow morning," said Linda.

"I'll clear my schedule and be waiting outside my office building," responded Ham.

CHAPTER 13
VENI, VIDI, VICI

I came, I saw, I conquered

Agent Linda Carter picked up Ham in her tan Ford Taurus. (What else? Has any federal agent seen on TV driven anything but a tan Ford Taurus?) They drove to the Philadelphia airport in relative silence, engrossed in their own thoughts. They were heading for a USAir commuter flight to Louisville, where they would rent a car and then drive fifty miles to Rancho Arabia. A Saudi sheikh named Abu Ben Gazar owned the horse farm.

Ben Gazar was a known acquaintance of Evan Stoner. In his role as a horse owner, Stoner had visited the Saudi approximately once a year for the last ten years, ostensibly to discuss breeding and purchasing of horses. Agent Carter and Ham were not going there to watch stallions mount mares, however. The Saudi connection, plus the events involving Ham and his wife with a series of Middle Eastern bad men, was too convenient. Neither Ham nor Agent Carter believed in those kinds of coincidences.

Besides, Agent Carter told Ham, she had had picked up a whiff of info that possibly linked Stoner as a NOC (no overt cover) to the CIA. A sort of courier of intel between a moderate Saudi, with family connections in Riyadh, and the CIA, as improbable as that sounded. She could neither confirm nor deny the connection, mainly because of the stovepipe mentality of the CIA toward the FBI (despite the Patriot Act). Her suspicions, however, along with Ham's innate curiosity, had convinced him to accompany her on this exploratory journey.

After having arrived at the Louisville airport, Agent Carter rented a tan Taurus (again!). One hour later, they drove up to the white arched gate with a logo of crossed Arabian swords mounted over a sign. In English, written in pseudo Arabic fashion, was "Rancho Arabia."

A dark-complexioned man, in a standard civilian security guard uniform, approached and asked in unaccented English what their business was at the "Rancho." Agent Carter flashed her credentials and explained that they had come to talk to "the sheikh" and had made a previous appointment. She wanted to be sure that the sheikh would be in country and at his ranch at the time of their visit. The armed guard consulted a handheld device and, after being satisfied of the legitimacy of Agent Carter and Ham's appointment, opened the gates to the farm.

The Taurus had to clear one more security gate, which opened slowly outward, but the passengers did not have to undergo another interrogation by the second security guard who was standing and holding a small wireless telephone, with a handgun holstered on his hip.

Ham and Agent Carter marveled at the sight before them. Acres and acres of magnificent bluegrass pastures covered the horizon; flowers and fountains dotted the landscape along the white stone driveway that seemed to go on for miles. Areas of the pastures were fenced off with miles of bright white fencing containing magnificent horses of all shapes and colors.

"I sure wish I had the fencing contract for this place," quipped Ham.

"I'd be happy with the grass-cutting job," answered Carter.

To the right of their path, mares and foals gamboled in the sunshine. To the left, dozens of magnificent stallions stamped and snorted. A few men in overalls were in the fenced-in areas riding on tractors, spreading hay bales, or collecting manure.

Coming over a small hill, the white stone path dipped into a valley that contained four or five red-tile-roofed buildings, all maintained to such perfection that they appeared to be out of an advertisement for a Middle Eastern or Mediterranean playground for the rich and famous.

One building stood out from this perfection. It was large, decorated with colored tiles about the entrance, and sat next to an Olympic-size swimming pool, which itself was surrounded by a tiled pool deck on which sat two dozen expensive deck chairs and umbrella tables. This was the owner's house, and that's where Ham and Carter headed, parking between the house and a magnificent fountain that was surrounded by a garden that brought Eden to the mind of Ham.

A man and a woman exited from the house and stood smiling as Linda and Ham left the car. Both were dressed in jeans and long-sleeved, plaid shirts. The woman was about Linda's height and also blonde. The man was the same height as the woman, with long, well-groomed, dark hair and a Van Dyck beard and mustache. Both were smiling widely with bright white dentition that would make a toothpaste company jealous.

"Welcome to Rancho Arabia! This is my wife, Jackie," the man said in Oxonian English as he indicated the woman standing to his right. "And I am Abu Ben Gazar, but my friends call me Abe, and I want you two to be my friends." The tanned, or dark-complexioned, man reached out his hand to Linda and then to Ham.

"Why, thank you for the nice greeting," Linda responded while offering her credentials to the man who called himself Abe.

"I am Agent Linda Carter, from the Federal Bureau of Investigation, and this is Dr. Marks, a forensic orthopedic surgeon from Philadelphia."

"Please, call me Ham," Ham said with a smile.

Linda continued. "As you know from my telephone call, we are here to talk to you about your business relationship with attorney Evan Stoner, who died recently."

"Oh, yes, I was so very sorry to hear about Evan's death. Before we get into such details, however, I would like to offer you the hospitality of Rancho Arabia. Won't you come in and have some fruit juice? You must be parched after your long drive." The sheikh indicated the entrance to his home with his outstretched hand.

Linda and Ham entered the house, with Jackie holding open the elaborately decorated door.

The inside of the house was just as magnificent, and elaborate, as the outside. The individual rooms were tiled with only strategically spaced areas of white plaster showing. Each room was entered through a tiled archway. The tiled floors were covered in various areas by ornate carpets. Adorning the plaster portions of the walls were spectacular paintings of individual horses with their names on the frames in both English and Arabic.

One room served as a dining area and the table was set with glasses, plates, crystal pitchers containing cold juices, and platters of fresh fruit and sweet baked goods.

"Please, help yourself," Jackie said as she gestured toward the table.

Linda and Ham did as they were bid, and while drinking their juice and munching on the sweet cookies they observed the rest of the house. Next to the dining area was an office with computers and a bank of video screens, which flashed from one scene to the next. Two women and a man sat at desks in front of the screens. Through another arch, the house seemed to go on forever—arch after arch, one magnificent room after another.

The sheikh, "Abe," indicated the office space. "We can monitor the entire farm from this room, via video cameras that are placed at various locations throughout the five hundred acres. You see, we have to maintain the well-being of all our mares and foals, and we can't let our stallions get into trouble either. We have seven hundred very expensive animals under our care here, not including the dogs and cats, of course." Abe chuckled. "And we have only a full-time staff of twenty, so we need the cameras to focus our attention on where the work needs to be done. Our headman even has a wireless camera that can send pictures back to this office from any particular area of concern."

The sheikh continued. "Before our important conversation about Evan Stoner begins, Jackie would love to take you on a short tour of the farm. Would you like that?"

Linda and Ham smiled and nodded and made muffled comments like "Oh, yes!" and "Of course!"

"Fine," said Abe. "I will meet you back here in our conference room after your tour."

The tour, on foot, took about forty-five minutes. Jackie escorted Ham and Linda through the various buildings where horse-breeding operations took place. They were fascinated by the concept of the teaser stallion whose only job was to get the mares excited, preliminarily for the big stallions to do their duty. And duty they did, up to a dozen times a day. This concept had Ham and Linda both shaking their heads at the prowess of the equine reproductive force.

"Do the stallions all belong to you and Abe?" Ham asked.

"No," Jackie answered in her unaccented English, which both Linda and Ham assumed was a product of her American upbringing. "We own a part of all the animals along with many others, such as Mr. Stoner. We receive a fee from each successful mating. The foals belong to the owners of the mares, including ourselves. We care for the animals and train them mainly for racing."

"Where does the connection to Saudi Arabia come in?" Linda queried.

"Well, Abe will often import Arabian stock to improve bloodlines," Jackie answered. "He visits his homeland two or three times a year for such purposes."

The walking tour continued through most of the buildings housing mares with foals and magnificent stallions, their coats shining and their nostrils flaring. Barely a stalk of straw was out of place. And the few men and women tending to the animals either kept the area neat as a pin or went about their animal husbandry work with determination and efficiency.

Ham noted, as he had been informed, the presence of dozens of mounted video cameras, some fixed and some able to be manipulated side to side and up and down from a central station. Occasionally, he would see a monitoring station tucked behind a stall, with several flickering screens, but never in such profusion as he had seen in the main house.

As they exited from the fourth building, Jackie pointed to the men in the pastures and explained that they were gathering manure.

"That's an onerous job," Ham commented.

"Not at all," Jackie replied quickly. "The ranch makes a small fortune selling manure for fertilizer to the farmers in Kentucky, particularly mushroom growers."

Linda and Ham first raised eyebrows and then turned down corners of their mouths almost simultaneously. Jackie laughed and then said, "I think we should return to the main house now, unless you have any more questions."

"No, thank you for the tour," Linda said.

Ham murmured, "Yes, thank you."

The trio entered the main house and moved to a conference room where Abe sat at a large, carved, wooden table. Jackie excused herself, and Abe rose to greet Linda and Ham. Abe handed both visitors crimson baseball caps with crossed Arabian swords above two gold, embroidered letters with "RA" in an Arabic font.

"Something to remember your visit by," Abe stated.

"Why, thank you, Abe, but I don't think either Ham or I will ever forget this visit, right Ham?"

"Absolutely right," Ham answered. "This place is magnificent."

"Thank you, Ham. Now what can I do for you two in regards to Evan Stoner? Please, sit down and tell me."

Linda began the conversation, with Ham as a silent onlooker. She explained Stoner's less than common deadly surgical outcome, Ham's position as the forensic orthopedic expert who was asked to investigate the circumstances of Stoner's death for a defense malpractice firm, and several of the dangerous "incidents" involving Ham and a Middle Eastern connection. She never approached the subject of Stoner being a NOC but did make the connection between Stoner and the Middle East, through Rancho Arabia, quite clear.

Abe looked puzzled at first. And then, after a long intake of breath, stated, "I am astounded that there is any Arabic connection involved in these attacks. And for these, I apologize to you, Dr. Marks, for all of Arabia. But I do not see any possible connection in your story to Rancho Arabia."

Linda was about to gradually approach the matter of Stoner collecting intel from the farm when a loud report was heard in the background. And then a second and a third. Linda was suddenly alert. "That sounds like gunfire," she announced.

At the same moment, a security guard cried out from his monitoring station in the next room, "Sheikh, Sheikh, you'd better come and see this! Something terrible has just happened at the gate! Someone is shooting at the guards!"

Abe, Linda, and Ham moved quickly into the monitoring room and stood behind the guard who was adjusting the screen. What they saw on the colored screen made their mouths drop. A small white truck with an open bed was barreling down the white stone path. In the back, Ham could see, were two men with their heads and faces wrapped in checkered kaffiyeh. They were brandishing automatic weapons.

"Play back the tape!" Abe ordered.

The security guard twisted a few dials and tapped a few keys on the monitor keyboard. A scene straight out of the streets of Baghdad, or perhaps Riyadh, erupted on the screen. The three onlookers stared with open mouths as the white truck barreled through first the outer gate and then the second gate with the masked men in the rear of the truck firing their weapons and felling the two guards who were taken completely by surprise.

"Call 911!" the sheikh shouted to the women in the office. "Tell the police that we have been invaded by masked gunmen who have killed our security guards. If they don't believe you, let them listen to the audio track of the videotape."

Linda, who took exactly thirty seconds to get her mind into FBI battle readiness, turned to the sheikh and asked calmly, "Do you have any weapons here in the house?"

"Why yes, I have two hunting rifles and a shotgun."

"Why don't you bring them in here with ammunition," Linda stated matter-of-factly.

She then spoke to Jackie, who had just entered the room, and Ham. "Have either of you ever fired a gun?"

Jackie replied that she had often gone hunting with the sheikh and that one of the hunting rifles was actually hers.

"I have a sharpshooter's badge from my army days. Does that count?" Ham replied.

"You bet!" Linda said. And then turning to the security guard and the women in the office, she said, "Please, all of you stay calm. I want you to firmly, but not loudly, call out where each one of the bad guys is as you spot them on your monitors, okay?"

"Okay," they all said in unison as they pulled their chairs up to the bank of monitors and adjusted the screens for clarity and focus.

"Where is the headman with the wireless camera?" Linda asked.

"There he is," said one of the women pointing to a monitor. "He's in the stallion building."

"Can you contact him by phone?"

"Yes," one of the terrified women said.

"Well, do that. Tell him what's going on and have him get all of the employees he can safely under cover. Also tell him to keep his camera rolling so we can have some mobile intelligence as to the whereabouts of the gunmen."

At that moment, the sheikh returned and laid out the three weapons and the ammunition on the carved wooden desk that sat at one end of the room. Linda moved over to the desk and expertly checked the weapons, loading each and making sure the safety was off.

"These weapons are loaded and ready to fire, so be very careful how you handle them. Abe and Jackie, why don't you take your hunting rifles and ammunition and set up at windows at each side of this building. I'll take the shotgun, and Ham, you take my weapon. Remember the safety is off. You have fifteen shots, and here are two more clips for you." Linda produced the weapon and the ammunition from behind her back.

"They're breaking off of the path and heading for the first building!" the guard shouted.

"Don't shout!" Linda remonstrated. "But keep the information coming. Ham, you get to the back of the house in case they decide to come in from there. And all of you, don't worry about hitting anything. If you see any one of them—I counted four men—just fire. The surprise that we have weapons should keep them ducking for cover. Again, if you see one of them, let the rest of us know."

A shotgun blast and the acrid smell of cordite interrupted Linda's instructions.

"Who fired?" she queried.

"I did," the sheikh's wife said in a calm manner. "I saw one of them approaching the house from the stable. He ducked back into the building after I fired."

"Good. That should keep them talking among themselves for a while," Linda stated matter-of-factly.

Two more shots rang out, one a shotgun blast and one a round from Linda's gun in Ham's hand. At the same time, several sirens began to shriek as four or five state police cars roared onto the property. They stopped in a cloud of dust, with the police troopers setting up behind the doors of their vehicles. Bulletproof vests on, they fired their own powerful weapons at the masked terrorists who were running between the horse farm buildings.

Very quickly, the masked men jumped into their vehicle and were roaring across the pastures, knocking down fences as they fled. The police vehicles, all except one, pursued the open truck with sirens blaring.

"Is everyone inside all right?" asked one of the police officers.

"Yes, we're fine," Linda answered, taking out her badge and identifying herself to the state policeman.

As the dust settled and heart rates returned toward normal, everyone sat around the headquarter house where they drank juice, ate cookies, and answered questions posed by the interviewing officer.

"Agent Carter, what in your opinion were they after?"

Linda didn't hesitate for a moment. "I think they were after us, Dr. Marks and myself, and when I get back to my field office in Philly I'll confirm that and inform you of my findings."

"Fine," said the officer. "We ought to have them under arrest shortly. After all, where can they go?"

"More to the point," said the sheikh, "where did they come from?"

"We'll have that information for you shortly, and we'll definitely let you know," said the state trooper as he collected his notes and left the premises.

Linda and Ham said their good-byes and apologized for bringing near disaster down on the sheikh's horse paradise.

Ham slept most of the way back to the airport, his violent dreams causing him to jerk several times in his seat belt.

CHAPTER **14**

GAUDEAMUS IGITUR

Let us rejoice

Clink-clink, clink-clink. The four champagne glasses clinked together in the small private room off of the main dining room of the Four Seasons Hotel, arguably the most expensive dining setting in Philadelphia.

"Gaudeamus igitur," exclaimed Ham to his wife, Agent Linda Carter, and Sam Broder, their host for this occasion.

"Does that mean you want another drink?" Broder asked.

"No, no, no," said Ham as he chuckled. "It means, 'Let us rejoice!' Congratulations to us all for our part in this medico-legal adventure."

"Well, you all certainly deserve thanks and praise for all that you went through during this case. And this little dinner is the least my firm can do for you after you saved our clients, Dr. Miller, the university hospital, and the HMO from possible multimillion-dollar verdicts against them."

"You're the one who deserves the credit by getting the judge to have the case thrown out of court," Ham said.

"It certainly wasn't difficult once we got the judge to listen *in camera* to the evidence that Linda brought us," Broder said with somewhat misplaced humility. "And then your finding of the cause of Stoner's death, Ham, was the topper."

"Not to be a party pooper here," Linda said with a serious visage despite the joviality of the occasion, "but I want to remind you all that what we say here about the conclusion of this case has to go no further than this room. Agreed?"

"Agreed," the rest of the party said in unison.

"After all, we don't want another Secretary Armitage incident to come out of this party," Linda said wryly. To which all gave a short guffaw.

"All right, now that we have all pledged our allegiance to the FBI and CIA, why don't you fill us in on all the details of what happened after you and Ham left Kentucky?" Broder invited.

"Okay," Linda said, and then she took a deep breath and started in with her tale.

"After Ham and I left Kentucky, I received a report that the Kentucky State Police had rounded up all the bad guys at a dude ranch that they were occupying outside of Louisville. Very few dudes, but a lot of Middle Eastern gentlemen, coming and going, according to neighbors. A number of shots were exchanged, but no one was hurt, thank goodness. The bad guys decided not to head for Paradise right then.

"It turned out that this was an Al Qaeda cell. Most of the men were from Saudi Arabia and had been in the country for many months. They had stirred the interest of the FBI, CIA, and Homeland Security, who were all watching from a distance, but the action of the Kentucky State Police brought them all together in a hurry.

"It must have been quite a colorful crowd! All those windbreakers with differing letters on the back. Anyhow, The Patriot Act scored again. All stovepipes came down, and the agencies worked together remarkably. As it turned out, this particular cell was tasked to take down the sheikh, at his ranch, along with Stoner the next time he visited. Ham's intervention in the case, even as a medical forensic investigator, put him right in their sights, as he found out on several occasions.

"At that point in time, they had already taken care of attorney Stoner at the hospital and they could not afford to have Ham figure out their plot. Stoner, it turned out, wasn't such a bad guy after all. He had been operating as a NOC for the CIA for a number of years. That's an agent, or informant, for the CIA with no overt cover. He was what he was. A rich malpractice lawyer with an interest in horseflesh.

"His visits to horse breeders in Saudi Arabia, and his connection with the sheikh in Kentucky, offered him the opportunity to gather and pass on information concerning Middle Eastern terrorism that was of immense value to the CIA. Al Qaeda found this out and planned to do away with Stoner well before he entered the hospital for his operation.

"Ham's and his wife's run-in with Mr. Said were part of the aftermath of this plan.

"Incidentally, the FBI picked up Mr. Said at the Philadelphia airport. He had a ticket to Louisville. Once he learned that the Kentucky cell had been rounded up, he was very cooperative about his role in the plot. Trying to be a big shot, I suppose.

"It turned out that his wife was trained as a paralegal and worked in Mr. Broder's office. That's how they got all of their advanced information about Ham."

"Really sorry about that, Ham," Broder said sheepishly.

Ham grinned.

"This is where Ham comes into the picture again," Linda said. "Ham, why don't you take it from here?"

"Okay, Linda," Ham said, putting down his champagne. "Mr. Said, trained as an orderly in Kentucky and elsewhere, was tasked to actually carry out the job of killing Stoner. He entered Stoner's hospital room postoperatively, with little difficulty since he actually was an orderly, and injected a small but lethal amount of ricin into Stoner's IV while he slept. Death was almost instantaneous.

"Ricin is a deadly concentration of a common plant, the castor bean, used in making castor oil, a perfectly harmless and very useful drug. Once I learned of this action, I immediately notified my friend, Pete Gross, the head of pathology at the university hospital. He revisited the toxicology specimens that were taken at the time of Stoner's autopsy and was able, with some difficulty, to detect very small amounts of ricin in several specimens.

"It was this objective evidence that convinced the judge that there was murder here, not malpractice. The judge, in turn, convinced Mrs. Stoner's attorney to withdraw all the suits against the multiple defendants. The judge explained that if they didn't do this, they would be liable for a charge of abuse of process if they continued the suits without a legitimate probable cause."

"So Stoner wasn't quite the bastard that he made himself out to be, was he?" queried Ruth Marks.

"He was a bastard all right, but his heart was softer than his liver," Sam Broder contributed. "In his will, he gave a multimillion-dollar gift to the university law school. They're going to create a building with his name on it. The rest of his money went to his two wives and his kids. He even gave gifts to his partner Mathews, his pilot, his horse trainer, his boat captain, and, believe it or not, to his ex-sister-in-law."

"Did that satisfy his present wife? And did she go off with the pilot?" Ham asked.

"That was quite a story, wasn't it?" Broder said. "It's a good thing we had such a terrific investigator to find out all the dirt on the players involved in this drama. But Mrs. Stoner had it figured all wrong. The pilot was married and had three kids—he quietly went back to Momma.

"Mrs. Stoner is anything but satisfied with her inheritance. She has hired a new lawyer and is suing the estate and her former lawyer, Mathews, who it turns out knew that Stoner had hidden assets that he didn't declare at the time of the divorce settlement. This lady is out for blood money!"

"Well, I guess that's to make up for her 'loss of consortium' award, which she failed to get," Linda said, half in jest.

"Don't laugh," Broder replied. "She was asking for five million dollars for 'loss of consortium,' not that she suffered from much of a lack of consortium, as it turns out."

"I certainly hope that this case teaches you a lesson, Ham—to look out for bad situations that Sam may get you into in the future," Ruth Marks admonished. She looked at both Ham and Sam Broder.

"Per aspera ad astra," Ham replied. "Only through difficulty can one reach the stars."

Before Ruth Marks could respond to that ambiguous remark, the shrimp cocktail was served.

A "C" CHANGE

Chapter 1

Et Tu, Brute?

Even you, Brutus

I love the Roman Forum. I've visited here four or five times in my sixty-three years, and each time I get another thrill. I pretend I'm a senator in ancient Rome strolling past the law courts and acknowledging the House of the Vestal Virgins, with several of the sacred ladies sunning themselves in the Garden of Statues. I approach the rostrum in front of the Senate building and either prepare to give a speech of my own to the senators and countrymen who congregate nearby or listen intently as Cicero speaks. I'm wearing my flowing white toga with a purple sash, just like the other senators who are preparing to enter the Senate.

Then the whole picture crashes before my eyes. At six feet two (I've lost an inch with the passing of years), balding, and weighing in at 230 pounds, I look like a gift-wrapped Michelin Man! But I still love the Roman Forum.

My wife, Ruth Ann Marks, MD, has left me on my own for a few hours as she strolls through Ferragamo's at the foot of the Spanish Steps. She's been to Rome a few times herself. She's a hardworking pediatrician with a small private practice at a hospital in Bryn Mawr in suburban Philadelphia. But her real love is her research work on cystic fibrosis. She runs a large laboratory and has a number of National Institutes of Health research grants. So ordinarily she has to be dragged kicking and screaming away from her rats and mice to take a vacation like the one we are on now. But I had recently concluded a big medico-legal forensic case, which was not only stressful to me (it even involved my participation in a gun battle with Arabic terrorists) but also to Ruth. She was carjacked by one of the terrorists. She didn't know that at the time but found out later, and that was enough to scare her away from her lab for a few weeks of R & R. Besides, she has a good *rat man* who cares for the animals. She calls him on the cell phone on a daily basis.

I hailed a cab at the Forum ticket gate. It's not always easy to hail a cab in Rome—even if you speak Italian, which I don't. Occasionally, Yiddish helps, since the cab drivers and most of the tchotchke sellers in Rome seem to be *lonsmen*. This driver understood "Grande Hotel," and after ten minutes of hair-raising, almost bumper-car driving through the impossible Roman traffic, I was dropped off at the portico of the hotel.

After figuring out the cab fare in Euros—what was it? 1.4 to the dollar or 1.4 dollars to the Euro?—and the tip, I exited the crash vehicle. Whatever the cost, it was certainly easier figuring it out than the cost of things in lire, like the last time I was here, which was twenty years ago. Fourteen hundred to the dollar. You had to be an idiot savant to figure the cost of things.

The Grande Hotel is really quite grand. It's completely in line with a number of first-class hotels in Rome that are hidden away among the ancient building fronts—like some camouflage that hides their magnificence from the Huns or the Goths. Or perhaps from the poor Romans who would be envious of the way rich visitors live in their ancient city while they, in many cases, still live like the Roman *populus* of Caesar's time. The Roman municipal administrators handle this unevenness in living quarters by reminding Romans of the ancient and undying love for them—as emblazoned on every municipal sewer lid: "SPQR." The Senatus Populusque Romanus. The Senate and the Roman People Forever—in the sewers, for heaven's sake.

Anyway, the Grande Hotel, as I said, is quite grand. I picked up the key to Ruth's and my suite, upgraded by American Express. That platinum card is good for something, I guess. With the little bit of overseas traveling that Ruth and I do during any one year, I have to squeeze every bonus I can from the extra three hundred bucks I pay for this fancy charge card. I did get an upgraded suite on the ship that would take us on our medico-legal conference as well, and I'm looking forward to staying in that "luxury" space after we board the ship tomorrow.

The hotel suite was spectacular, with fine wood paneling, mosaic tile floors, and beautiful oil paintings on the walls. The two bathrooms actually looked too good to do one's normal ablutions in—but for two days I could get used to it without feeling guilty toward the hoi polloi who were not able to enjoy such luxury. After all, what good is it to be a Republican if you can't have a few guilty pleasures?

Ruth was taking a nap—exhausted after her shopping spree. Six pairs of shoes in their Ferragamo's boxes, with the lids off, sat on the bench at the foot of the bed. I had to laugh silently when I thought of the tale of how much money she saved by "buying in bulk" here in Rome. But after all, it was her money.

I washed up for dinner in the Roman bath they called a bathroom, thinking of the tale told to me by the bellhop that Richard Burton and Elizabeth Taylor stayed in the same suite while they were making the movie *Cleopatra*. I figured Burton would have had both of the beautiful wood-paneled closets and the medicine cabinets filled with booze, while I just had Pepsodent toothpaste and a second pair of shoes in mine.

I then waited a long, long, long time for Ruth to ready herself for dinner. It really wasn't a great hardship since the magnificent Anthony and Cleopatra Suite also sported a fifty-inch, flat-screen HD TV, which allowed me to watch Fox News while waiting with a Diet Coke and mini pretzels on the side.

Ruth and I walked around the corner from the hotel to a *trattoria* (I guess that means "little restaurant" in Italian) and sat down at a checkered-tablecloth-covered table to enjoy the local ambience. Ruth asked me, "What would you like to eat, dear?"

The waiter mumbled something unintelligible in Italian to us. My mother may have been a classicist and known six or seven ancient and modern languages, but, unfortunately, that seemed not to rub off on me. I thought, *A nice little steak filet with a baked potato and asparagus would do nicely*, but I said, "What on earth are those green and white things hanging over our heads? And am I supposed to eat one of those giant bolognas hooked to the ceiling beams?"

To which Ruth replied, "Never mind, dear. I'll order for you."

And she did, and I ate it. And I survived.

On the walk back to the hotel, I reviewed the upcoming cruise with Ruth. I said, "I'll be tied up in meetings most mornings, but we'll tour in the afternoons."

"That's all right, dear. I plan to work out and learn mahjong," Ruth replied.

"The room should be nice with all of our upgrades."

"As long as the bags get there, I'll be happy," Ruth countered.

With that, we reached the Grande and proceeded to bed with the ghosts of Anthony and Cleopatra.

CHAPTER 2
EUROPA STAR

We rose to a beautiful June morning in Rome, ate breakfast in our suite, washed, dressed, and entered our air-conditioned Mercedes limo for the ride to Civitavecchia, where our ship *Europa Star* was docked for the embarkation for our trip. I figured if we are going to go for broke, we might as well go all the way—using up a small portion of our kids' inheritance since they had been pampered enough up to now.

This was Ruth and my "C" change. That sounded like a very clever ploy—you know, a sea change on a ship, on the *sea*. But that was one of my pet peeves. I always interpreted *sea change*—normally interpreted as a conditional change in the wind and waves of the sea from calm to violent—as a "C" change. That is, a change in direction 180 degrees—starting to go one way and ending up going in the exact opposite direction like writing a capital "C." So this double entendre had Ruth and me going from landlubberly, hardworking, medical providers, to sea-going tourists bound for ten days of enjoyment without a care in the world—or so we thought.

Of course I was taking a course of lectures on medico-legal medicine. But in reality, that was just a getaway excuse. Both Americans and Europeans gave the lectures. They were interesting but not earth shaking in their content. There was no note-taking requirement or seminars or tests. The thirty to fifty docs and paramedical and medico-legal participants were all planning to have a good time after the lectures, which were all given in the a.m. There would be booths outside of the lecture hall with relevant books and journals for sale as well as interesting medical and legal products for sale by some of the more entrepreneurial international participants. In other words, I was expecting to learn a little, but in an interesting and tax-free environment, and spend the rest of the time as a plain old European tourist with Ruth.

For the heck of it, I planned to visit the ship's infirmary and offer my orthopedic services to the ship's medical officer, who was probably a general practitioner who was basically along for the ride. My volunteering duty wasn't going to get me a bigger tax deduction, but it was going to provide me with the old saw of the shoemaker mending his lasts. In other words, it would make me feel better if I had some sort of practical orthopedic connection to this trip.

It took over an hour to reach the ship, albeit in the lap of luxury, but I was hungry, again, when we reached the dock. Having prepared ahead of time for a smooth transition from land to shipboard life, Ruth and I signed in, had our pictures taken, and were escorted, glass of champagne in hand, to our suite in rapid order. The persistent semifrown on Ruth's face only disappeared completely when the steward opened our cabin door and she saw all of our luggage safely delivered and set out on luggage racks. Our butler (butler!) introduced himself and offered to help unpack, a service that Ruth only partially accepted. No one likes to have anyone see the underwear in his or her luggage.

Anthony and Cleopatra never rode in the *Europa Star*, but if they had then they would have been in our suite. It was at the stern of the ship with a magnificent viewing veranda and a built-in hot tub. The suite indoors included a bedroom with a big bathroom, a dining area, and a living room with a giant flat-screen TV. It also had a second bathroom, which immediately became mine, Ruth having commandeered the large one. Ruth was happy, and if she was happy I was happy.

I finally convinced Ruth (or perhaps my loud borborygmus did the trick) that her "big boy" needed feeding, so off we went to explore and restore.

The ship had five complete restaurants, a luncheon buffet, and a coffee shop. We chose the buffet and, after making some very difficult choices, we ate. After our meal we wandered about the ship. We stopped outside of the conference room to be used for the medico-legal lectures and I showed Ruth where I would be spending my mornings for the next week.

"Looks comfortable," Ruth said.

"Hmmmm," I said, but I thought, *I just can't wait for my butt to go numb sitting in those comfortable seats for three hours.* Chastened with that thought, we headed back to our luxurious suite. We finished unpacking. I had taken the valet up on his unpacking abilities, and he had done a much better job than I could have done. I showered and dressed for dinner and then sat down in front of the large flat-screen TV to watch Fox News and do some catching up on my computer, which just loved the onboard Wi-Fi system.

I had plenty of time. Ruth finished unpacking and preparing herself for dinner by eight p.m. We watched the ship depart from Civitavecchia on the Italian coast from our veranda, sipping the wine and munching on the hors d'oeuvres supplied by Roger, our butler. Before heading for open-seating dinner, I suggested to Ruth that we visit the infirmary so that I could introduce myself to the ship's doctor. We took the elevator down lower than I had ever been on a cruise ship. We stepped off the elevator and entered a stainless-steel empire. Everything was made of stainless steel: floors, walls, cabinets, tables. And it was a huge room.

In the middle of this shiny world sat a less-than-shiny gentleman. He was bald, dumpy, and short but with a pleasant personality that shone through the gleam. He was wearing a white uniform with shoulder epaulets bearing three golden bars. The man introduced himself. "Hello, I'm Dr. Rosenbaum. What can I do for you folks?"

"Dr. Rosenbaum, I'm Dr. Ham Marks, and this is my wife, Dr. Ruth Marks. I'm an orthopedic surgeon, and I'm here to participate in the medico-legal conference. I thought I'd just come down here and introduce myself and offer my services, in case you ever needed them during the cruise."

"Why that's very kind of you, Dr. Marks. I'm a general practitioner from Altoona, Pennsylvania, and I must say I'm a bit rusty on orthopedic procedures, so I welcome your offer. Here, let me just write down your name and cabin number, just in case."

"Dr. Ham Marks, suite 1036," I said. "But, please, just call me Ham."

"All right, Ham. I'm Ben. Why don't you just look around and make sure that all the equipment you might need is here. If not, I'm sure I can get it sent in."

"Right," I said.

I began to check some of the stainless-steel and glass cabinets, which appeared to have all the material I would need to treat any orthopedic conditions that I could conceive of as occurring on the high seas. "Looks like it's all here, Ben."

"Good. Thanks for coming down, Ham. And here's hoping I never have to give you a call. Nice to meet you, Mrs. . . . . I mean *Dr.* Marks." He reached out to shake Ruth's hand.

"A pleasure, Dr. Rosenbaum. Beautiful place you have here," she said, not really knowing what else to say.

I shook Ben's hand and Ruth and I backed out of the clinic. We made our way back to the dining room.

Dinner was a delight. A daily menu was provided, but in reality we could order anything at all—cooked to our own specifications. Elephant was not included. You know, the joke about not killing an elephant for just one steak. Well, anyway, I know the joke, and I smiled. The waiters, busboys, sommelier, and head and assistant maitre d' were trained superbly for maximum service. They hailed from everywhere: Great Britain, Bulgaria, Romania, Ukraine, Russia, with just a smattering of Americans and Far Easterners. The multiple languages made the place feel like a traveling UN, with delicious smells. Ruth felt right at home, using her ability to converse in six or seven languages at one sitting. I, on the other hand, got by with a smile and a pointing finger.

We ate at a table for two, but that was just to get the opening night's lay of the land. We fully expected to eat with some of the doctors in the seminar for the rest of the trip.

We indulged in a postprandial drink at one of the dozen or so magnificent bars onboard, and then off we went to bed. The entertainment would still be there during the next eleven days, we felt, and I did have to get up early for the start of the conference.

CHAPTER 3

SUMMA CUM LAUDE

Highest honors

"Shoum, shoum, shoum." That's what I heard at Bulgarian secret police headquarters in Sofia. In your language, that means "chatter," information picked up by clandestine agents, on the Internet, or on telephone wiretaps—there are still plenty of those in my country as well as yours. Something was about to go down internationally. Whether on the land or sea or in the air, we did not know, but we were going to cover everything we could to protect the motherland.

I got the cushy job of covering the goings-on onboard the *Europa Star*. But then I deserved it. I was the "fair-haired boy" of the service. (How do you think I picked up all these American phrases?) I had spent three years in America getting a master's degree in pharmacology at Case Western Reserve University in Cleveland, Ohio, from 1990 until 1993. At the time, my brethren in the clandestine services of Bulgaria were getting their collective asses kicked out into the cold, cold Sofian winter.

It was the time of the conversion from the KGB style of operation to the new democratic Bulgarian DANS style: smaller, smarter, but just as dirty. You don't think that just because we were reduced in size by two thirds, and we were the protectors of the new *free* Bulgaria, that we were going to forget everything the Russians taught us.

But no more *umbrella* murders like we pulled off in 1978 when Francesco "Piccadilly" Gullino stabbed that disgusting defector Georgi Markov with a ricin-tipped umbrella as he walked across Waterloo Bridge in London. We even turned over to the Vatican all of the secret-service files we had collected on the Bulgarian who had helped the Turk who tried to assassinate Pope John Paul II in 1981, just to show how cooperative we had become in the new world order.

But enough of my defense of the new Bulgarian Secret Service. What am I doing here? My training in the United States gave me three valuable attributes as far as the DANS is concerned. Number one: I sound more like a Midwestern American than I do a Bulgarian. Two: my pharmacology degree, legitimately or not, allows me to call myself "Doctor," so I fit right in with the doctors who signed up for this medico-legal conference aboard the *Europa Star.*

The National Security Service, headquartered in the Ministry of Internal Affairs in our capital city of Sofia, has control over domestic law enforcement, including cases of international criminal activity, organized crime (Mafia), smuggling, political corruption, and illegal fascism or nationalist organizations. One of the most troubling illegal international activities involves the pharmaceutical industry. Industrial espionage, Mafia control, and smuggling of pharmaceutical products form a multibillion-dollar enterprise.

Pravda, that news source of truth and virtue, has reasonably proclaimed that the Mafia dominate the Russian pharmaceutical industry—and that would pertain as well to Ukraine and Bulgaria.

Putin, when he was in control in Russia, proclaimed that profits—mostly illegal profits—in Big Pharma surpass even illegal narcotic sales.

In any case, the possible involvement of Big Pharma, the Mafia, and criminal activity in the Bulgaria-Ukraine area of the world is why I was selected for this difficult assignment.

It's not all *playing doctor,* riding in a luxurious ocean liner, and eating and drinking like I never could in Bulgaria. Something didn't smell right to the bosses in the ministry so they decided to send their best man to find the source of the odor.

Obviously, no one knows who I am—except the ship's captain. I do carry a weapon: a small, thirty-eight-caliber Ruger semiautomatic pistol with a laser-targeting device, but I have promised the captain that my weapon will be locked in the cabin safe—except when I feel the need to carry it.

Now, I did not expect to uncover a cache of pharmaceuticals being smuggled to Russia, Turkey, Greece, or India. That's the job for the border agents. They find such treasures aboard trucks and buses daily at the Kalotina border in vehicles with Turkish, Bulgarian, and German license plates. At another border crossing near the Greek and Macedonian borders lies Blagoegrad, perhaps the ancestral home of Illinois's infamous governor. Blagoegrad is notorious as the gangster capitol of Bulgaria, and I've spent many a cold winter night on that border myself.

No. It was men, or women, and not material, that I was after on my twelve-day shipboard odyssey. I had dossiers on three of the doctors attending this conference—that's right, *dossiers*. We prepare for these assignments with everything that Interpol, Russia's FSB—formerly known as the KGB—and Google can come up with. I also had the boarding information, thanks to a cooperative captain, on all the other conference participants, as well as other cruise customers. The captain wanted no trouble aboard the *Europa Star*, and he just happened to be married to a lovely Bulgarian woman. Strange consequence, yes? He even supplied me with the personnel files on his crew and the international service persons. So I had a cabin full of files to keep me busy reading, which meant I would miss the nightly entertainment and barhopping. But then you can't have everything, even if you are Bulgaria's finest.

Oh, the third reason I was chosen for the job is that I was educated at St. Clement of Ohrid University of Sofia, Bulgaria's oldest and finest institute of higher education, and spent time abroad, so I know seven languages: Bulgarian, Russian, Ukrainian, English, Turkish, Greek, and some Rumanian. I was the smartest agent in the service, if I must say so myself, and the one most likely to turn up the source of the *shoum*, if it existed, aboard this ship.

My name is Simeon Markov, and I am no relation to the old defector. Markov just happens to be a common Bulgarian name. I'm nondescript. That is, I'm five feet nine, weigh just over 175 pounds, and have a slowly growing bald spot in the back of my otherwise black-hair-covered pate. I'm forty-eight years old, but I could just as well pass for thirty-eight or fifty-eight, if anyone were to attempt to guess my age. In other words, I don't exist.

But I do. And I can shoot out the eye of a bird in flight at twenty meters.

CHAPTER 4
SINE QUA NON

Without which there is nothing

I can't resist Danish pastries! Especially with cherry, or perhaps lemon centers. I know I shouldn't indulge, but I was hungry and that was all they offered, besides coffee and juice, at the preseminar breakfast at seven thirty in the morning. The classroom was at the back of the main deck, just next to the Danish pastries.

Outside of the room were booths—three or four of them—set up to command the attention of the participants during the break time. Each booth had a placard announcing the material that was to be demonstrated, including medical books, some of which were written by conference participants. For example, an AIDS book and material about US public health law as it pertained to the treatment of AIDS. And a booth with a well-designed billboard advertising a special product: Vanishe sea-foam cream. It was made from sea cucumber stem cells—of all things!—which got rid of unsightly pigmented senile keratoses that plague most of us after the age of fifty. Vanishe was apparently invented by one of the seminar participants, Boris Petrov, a doctor from Varna, Bulgaria.

I entered the "classroom," a well-lit room with windows overlooking the passing Mediterranean waves formed by the ship's wake. About fifty men and women sat in student chairs with a fold-down lap table that could be used for taking notes.

Most of the seminar participants, like me, had small sticky labels attached to their shirts or jackets announcing their name and region of origin. A few folks in the back rows had no labels. They had been encouraged to "come on in" and listen to the talks in order to fill up the room, but they would not get tax deductions and they would be looked upon with disapproval when they picked up a Danish and coffee.

The organizers of the course, several of whom were MDs and JDs (physicians and lawyers in one), sat up front with the participants. I had dealt with a number of MD-JDs in my forensic practice, and whenever I encountered such a dual professional I always thought about the joke pertaining to their group: the doctors that they dealt with thought that they "must be good lawyers" and the lawyers they dealt with always thought, *Ah well, they must be good doctors.*

Anyway, the organizers were handing out material to the "tagged ones," including a list of the participants, the names and backgrounds of the lecturers, along with the titles of their talks, and pencils, paper, and tickets to get more Danishes at break time. The organizers in the first row would introduce the lecturers and lead the question-and-answer sessions after the lectures. That is, if anyone stayed for the Q & A with the smell of warm Danishes wafting into the room.

I glanced at the list of lecturers as I squeezed myself into a student desk chair. It was an interesting group. At the very least, the geographical distribution was worth noting. There were docs from Utica, New York; Toms River, New Jersey; Odessa, Ukraine; and Varna, Bulgaria. Now there's worldwide distribution. There was even a Bulgarian named Markov with a degree in pharmacology from Case Western University in Cleveland.

Well, it was going to be fun trying to match the face with the country (without cheating by reading the sticky tag).

The lecture series began at eight o'clock. I must admit that I snoozed a bit, but I was wide-awake for a lecture on the legal aspects of caring for HIV patients. The lecture was given by a doctor trained in Odessa who was now on the Infectious Disease Service of the hospital of UCLA. So I crossed him off my "guess his origin" list. Ivan Shevenko was his name, and he had such a heavy Eastern European accent that his speech was difficult to understand. But his actual lecture was unintelligible. He first explained how viruses infect humans. But when it came to the legal ramifications regarding dealing with HIV-infected patients, his talk was nothing less than gibberish. I looked around the room to see if others were as perplexed as I was. Many were yawning or reading the day's news on the ship's version of the *Herald Tribune*. I couldn't figure out why he bothered to give such a terrible talk. If he were using his position on the faculty to get a free trip home for a visit, that would be one thing. But this ship's course was taking us nowhere near the Black Sea port of Odessa.

Oh, well. I was still going to get my tax write-off whether I understood his lecture or not.

At the conclusion of the morning lectures, we were given the opportunity to visit the booths outside of the lecture room. Some were manned by participants in the program; others were purely commercial exhibits.

There were several interesting books written by the docs at the seminar, and I flipped through a few, thinking, *Darn, I should have brought along a few dozen copies of my own books. Maybe I could have found a few takers here on the high seas. I certainly didn't reach best-seller status back on terra firma.*

The booth manned by the Ukrainian out of LA actually had some interesting information and statistics on AIDS treatment. It was as if a ghostwriter had created the written material and the *ghost* had given the lecture.

The most interesting booth, and the one surrounded by the most doctors (some of them still licking Danish lemon filling off of their fingers) was the booth giving information about the skin cream Vanishe. The Bulgarian doctor, Boris Petrov, who had invented the stuff, was an impressive-looking gentleman. He was a tall, well-built man with a full head of long white hair and a handlebar mustache and goatee. He spoke with a deep basso voice, but like his fellow faculty member from Ukraine his accent made it very difficult to understand him. Consequently, the doctors trying to hear his spiel were all grouped closely around him.

Apparently he had invented this product in the dermatology department of Varna Medical University and licensed it to a large Greek pharmaceutical company that had produced a first-class marketing display. The "secret" of Vanishe sea-foam cream was the culturing of and the extraction from sea cucumber (Holothuroidea) of their stem cells.

While the crowd around Petrov was straining to hear his answers to their questions, I was standing a bit behind the group and reading the very professional literature he was offering as a handout. It showed beautiful four-color photographs of before and after shots of the removal of very ugly, darkly pigmented lesions from the arms, chest, and backs of otherwise attractive patients after a series of applications of Vanishe. Very impressive.

The Greek company he had licensed his product to was called Olympias Products, Inc. and was headquartered in Macedonia, Greece. The classical background I inherited from my dear mother went into high gear. Olympias was the name of Alexander the Great's mother, the queen of ancient Macedonia. You remember the devilish woman played by Angelina Jolie in the movie.

Anyhow, the back page of the Olympias brochure also included some fine print concerning Vanishe sea-foam cream. Apparently it had also been found in some clinical trials to cure a cutaneous (skin) form of lymphoma known as mycosis fungoides. Now that would be big news, perhaps worth billions of dollars on the world market, if that turned out to be true.

The group around Dr. Petrov began to break up. The man directly in front of me was short, slim, and had a three-inch bald spot in the back of his head. As he turned to leave the display table, I noticed that his sticky tag said "Dr. Simeon Markov," the pharmacologist from Bulgaria and Cleveland, Ohio. I was about to cross him off my "match the face with the name" list, but he moved away quickly, and there was nothing particularly noticeable about his face. So I wasn't able to place a face check next to his name. Ah well, I'd see him again, I was sure, and I'd certainly recognize him by his bald spot.

I placed the Vanishe brochure in my pocket to show to Ruth. She would certainly know more about mycosis fungoides than I did.

I set out for the dining room to meet Ruth for lunch. The ship was docking shortly and Ruth and I were going to take a bus tour for the afternoon to Florence.

CHAPTER 5
MODO JOCABAR

I was only joking

No more lemon Danish! Please! I'd much prefer a bowl of borscht—with sour cream topping—but the likelihood of the doctors' conference serving that for breakfast was small to none.

I'd just return to my stateroom with a cup of tea to finish the analysis of the people on this trip who might possibly cause trouble. My room, by this time, looked like a workspace in the Library of Congress. Remember that I spent three years in Cleveland. Speaking of Cleveland, my job reminded me of the days I spent at Cleveland Stadium, watching the Indians battle for obscurity. You had to have a program to know the players.

My program was pasted all over the walls of my stateroom. I actually paid the stewards to stay out of my room. For the sake of hygiene, I allowed them to change my bedclothes once a week.

One wall had pictures of the relevant members of the ship's staff taped on, with the captain's data concerning each staff member's job and city and country of origin, and service record with this ship and with the line and with any other international company.

Another wall contained information, with pictures if available, of all of the ship's travelers with European backgrounds. The captain's list plus Google entries were included.

Finally, posted over my bunk, were the pictures and backgrounds of all the participants in the medico-legal conference, presenters as well as exhibitors and participants. Most of the professionals at the conference had Google entries, which were useful. I also looked up the institutions where they worked or trained.

Some list! I estimate there were 200 to 250 entries. I had to review all of them and then rate them as to a class of potential trouble. Class three—very unlikely to give me trouble. Class two—possibly, but not likely to give me trouble. Class one—suspicious characters.

I went over the data three or four times before I was satisfied with my classification, memorizing the data as I went along. Finally, my first-class list contained twenty-five names that were worth personal investigation on an ASAP basis.

An engineer by the name of Bergman hailed from the former East Germany. He was in a position to cause trouble in the engine room and I would have to pay him a visit—probably on his off time—to find out more about him.

A helmsman by the name of Rashov was from St. Petersburg and old enough to be a communist or perhaps a KGB plant. I would take the tour of the ship's helm, check name tags, and feel him out.

On the wait staff, a man from Bulgaria—named Boroshov—piqued my interest. He was older than the other waiters, who were in their twenties and thirties, and had been around tourist ships for about ten years. But disciplinary problems had kept him from being promoted. I would have to track him down and offer him a drink some night to see just what was on his mind.

A sommelier from Ukraine named Maria Mosenko would have to be questioned. She had transferred to the *Europa Star* just for this trip, after being on another ship in their line for four years.

Among the cruise participants, only three names stuck out. Two cruisers were from Bulgaria and one from Russia. The Bulgarians—Bohdan Ivanchuk and Andrij Babich—were definitely of interest. Both of them were big men over six feet tall and weighing over 250 pounds. They were both from Sofia, and although their occupations were listed as carpenters they both had records of minor criminal offenses, mostly battery and small-time B & E, according to my State Security sources. One wonders how they could afford this cruise and whether they had some ulterior motives. They definitely bore watching.

A traveler named Olga Alexandrova listed her city and country of origin as St. Petersburg, Russia. She was thirty-eight years old and listed her occupation as "homeowner." Right! The FBS report on her was much more interesting. First of all, she was the daughter of Russian General Alexander Borovich, a general officer in Russian intelligence who made a fortune gobbling up failed businesses. The businesses failed, of course, because the Russian government didn't like the owners' politics and closed them down, mainly by accusing the owners of failure to pay taxes.

Olga had no criminal record but had a reputation as a playgirl who, in her more sober moments, watched over a number of the general's businesses, including, interestingly, a multimillion-dollar pharmaceutical company. Well, I certainly had common interests to talk about with her. By reputation she was a major cougar, so I'd have to play my hand carefully with her. But it should be fun.

Among the participants in the medico-legal conference, there were three interesting men. Two were participants (speakers and exhibitors) and one was a medical doctor from the United States who was, as far as I could determine, just along for the ride—and the lemon Danish.

The first doctor was a dermatologist from Varna, Bulgaria. Boris Petrov was on the staff of the Medical University of Varna. Information on Dr. Petrov was easy to obtain from my DANS colleagues who keep complete records on just about every citizen of Bulgaria over the age of fourteen. He was speaking at the conference about patenting a new drug in Europe and Bulgaria in particular. And he was using his own invention, a cream apparently made from sea cucumber stem cells. *Hhmm*, sounded fascinating. Anyhow, his cream, which he calls Vanishe sea-foam cream, apparently did a great job of removing senile keratoses, the bane of existence for every vain white woman over the age of fifty-five. Sounded like a winner to me. Also, there were some rumbles that in clinical trials the drug had proven effective in treating mycosis fungoides—a form of cancer, which affected the skin.

The most interesting fact about the good Dr. Petrov and his cream was that he had licensed its production and distribution to a Greek or Macedonian company. That surely pissed off the commercial powers in Bulgaria and twisted the noses of big Russian pharma, which would love to get a hold of a product that had the potential to make billions for the motherland. Perhaps that's where Olga Alexandrova's interest came into the picture. I'd have to investigate that aspect further.

The second doctor participant of interest (at least to the Bulgarian secret police) was from Odessa. Ivan Shevenko was a specialist in infectious diseases. He trained at the Odessa State Medical University but emigrated to the United States and now taught at UCLA. His topic of interest was AIDS prevention, treatment, and the legal ramifications thereof. I didn't know where he fit into this puzzle, but I decided to have a conversation with him nonetheless.

Finally there was the doctor from Philadelphia. I've been to Philadelphia, and I like the city. But I could never figure out why they hadn't fixed the crack in their "Liberty Bell."

Dr. Ham Marks was an orthopedic surgeon. He apparently was interested in medico-legal forensics, which meant that he often stuck his nose in places where it didn't belong. He was a big man, but not tough looking. He spent a long time at the exhibit of Dr. Petrov's Vanishe cream. But more ominous was the fact that he took an interest in me. I could feel him staring at my bald spot. (I told you I had eyes in the back of my head.) Well, it should be easy enough to make friends with the good Dr. Marks.

CHAPTER 6
CAVEAT EMPTOR 2

Beware

It was a bit irritating getting up at six thirty in the morning, but Ruth and I had to shower, dress, and eat a light breakfast brought to the suite by our butler, before boarding our sightseeing bus in the port city of Livorno, Italy. We were headed for Florence. Really tough duty!

The bus took ninety minutes to reach Florence. We then toured the Accademia museum to see the magnificent statue of David by Michelangelo. Ruth and I were both impressed by the anatomic accuracy of the sculptor, although we both agreed that David's feet were too big.

The next stop was at the Piazza della Signoria, where the copy of the David statue resides outside of the City Hall next to the Uffizi Galleria. The weatherproof giant reproduction of the David statue fascinated us as we ate frozen gelato cones outside.

We crossed the Ponte Vecchio and explored the stalls selling everything from jewelry to crockery—all of it overpriced. We turned back to the left bank of the Arno River and headed on down to Harry's American Bar for an overpriced Coke and a BLT sandwich. But the ambience was great.

The final stop on our whirlwind tour of Florence was at the Piazza di Santa Croce, dominated by the magnificent church of Santa Croce where the remains of Michelangelo, Galileo, and Dante were said to reside. The piazza was another shopper's paradise.

This time, even Ruth bought some gold jewelry in a store strangely named Misuri, and some red leather gloves at Caesar's Leather Shop. The gold was my treat, but Ruth bought the gloves on her own.

Back on the bus, we took a swing around the magnificent Duomo (Santa Maria Church) with its world-famous, gilded bronze, carved doors.

Then off to the ship and some sleep. I awoke with Ruth poking me in the ribs with her elbow. *"Whaa?"* I said. To which she answered, "Did you notice the woman in the rear seat? Who is she?"

I twisted in my seat and peeked through the separation between the seat bodies. There, spread out on the large rear seat, amid large shopping bags carrying the names of the world's most luxurious stores—Gucci, Prada, Valentino, and Ferragamo's—was a striking blonde woman dressed to the nines and chattering away with one of the doctors, who was not with his wife.

"I don't know who she is, but I've seen her at some of the medical meetings," I said. "She's not a doctor, as far as I know. I've heard her called 'Olga,' and she talks like that Huffington woman—you know, with some sort of Slavic accent."

"Well, she sure knows how to capture the scene," said Ruth snidely.

"Yes, I guess she does," I said. And with that, we both fell back into our doze states.

That night, we had a wonderful dinner aboard ship. The waiters danced around us and gave the impression that we were in the dining room of the United Nations: French, German, and South African wait staff and a Russian sommelier. We retired to our suite with our tummies full and ready for a good night's sleep. I had more lectures early in the morning and we were off to Amalfi at midnight. We watched a rerun of the day's Fox News, and then went off to bed.

I was in the middle of making hospital rounds in my dreams when the hospital fire alarm went off. I was awake immediately and noted that the alarm bell was coming from the bedside telephone. Before picking up the receiver, I checked the alarm clock next to the phone. Three a.m.

"Hello, who is this?"

"Dr. Marks, this is Dr. Rosenbaum, the ship's doctor. So sorry to wake you up at this hour, but I've got a problem and I could use your help—since you offered."

"Sure thing, Doc. What can I do for you?" I said, assuming that I could answer his query and return to my dream state in short order.

"I've got a passenger here—a doctor, actually—who has received a rather significant traumatic injury to his lower leg, and I wonder whether you would be kind enough to come down to the infirmary and give me a hand with it."

"Sure. No problem, Doc. Give me about fifteen minutes to put my pants on and splash some water on my face and I'll be right down."

"Thank you, Dr. Marks," said a relieved Dr. Rosenbaum, who then hung up.

I explained the situation to Ruth, washed and dressed, and then headed down to Dr. Rosenbaum's stainless-steel bastion.

When I entered the shiny steel room, my eyes immediately fell upon a male patient who was bleeding from a wound in his left leg.

I nodded to Dr. Rosenbaum, who mouthed a silent, "Thank you!" and approached the patient. Instantly I recognized the white hair and white goatee. It was the Bulgarian doctor, Boris Petrov, who had invented Vanishe sea-foam cream.

"Dr. Petrov, what happened?" I asked as I examined the wound on his lower leg.

"I was assaulted," he said in his Bulgarian accent. "By two big men as I was walking on the deck."

"What were you doing out on the deck at that hour?" I asked in order to get the history straight.

"I am not a good sleeper, nor am I a good sailor. So I walk at night."

"Every night?" I asked.

"Yes, each night. I get tired, then I sleep."

"Well, how did your leg get injured?"

"As I say, these two big men . . . I could not see their faces. I think they wear masks, or at least dark makeup. They approach me and without a word force me to the railing. I think I am going over so I wrap my leg around a lower rail. In order to free my leg, they struck it against the railing many times. The pain was horrible, and I feared I would lose my grip. At that moment a passing passenger shouted out and the two men ran off."

I turned to Dr. Rosenbaum and asked, "What have you done for Dr. Petrov so far?"

"I've administered IM morphine for pain and tetanus toxoid and IM antibiotics prophylactically. I've elevated and cleansed the wound with

Betadyne—all before I called you. I also x-rayed the lower leg and ruled out fracture."

"Very good, Doctor. Dr. Petrov, you are very fortunate not to have suffered an open fracture. We would have had to get you off this ship and to a local hospital had that happened. But I think we can treat this wound onboard, if that's all right with you."

"Yes, please. I thank you for taking your time to treat me, Dr. Marks."

"No problem. Now let's take a look at this wound."

After a careful exam, including a vascular and neurological evaluation, I concluded that the good doctor had suffered a severe pretibial contusion and laceration, which had resulted in an open wound through the subcutaneous tissue down to the fascia.

"I think we should treat this wound in an open fashion," I said to Dr. Rosenbaum. "Sterile dressings, with multiple dressing changes, and Betadyne applications until the wound closes on its own. We should splint his leg from thigh to toes with a posterior splint held on loosely with an Ace bandage wrapped on with little or no tension. I think you should keep him here in the infirmary for the first few days with the leg moderately elevated. He will require hourly checks on his pedal pulses and a check on foot and toes sensation and motor power. Do you have an assistant who can do this, Doctor?"

"Oh, yes. There are two RNs who are assigned to the infirmary and I'll train them how to check the leg hourly for the first twenty-four hours. They can rotate eight-hour shifts."

"Is that all right with you, Dr. Petrov? Do you wish to call your wife or family member to come down so that we can talk to them?"

"No, no, no. Wife stay at home with children. I am here alone, so I do exactly as you say. Thank you."

Turning to Dr. Rosenbaum, I said, "The main reason to treat this wound open, and not suture it closed, is to avoid undue compression of the fascial compartment by swelling, which might cause a compartment syndrome and produce a loss of neuromuscular function due to vascular compromise."

"I understand, Doctor."

With that, I helped Dr. Rosenbaum apply a posterior plaster splint, checked the orders for the nurses, and, after a "Good luck" to both doctor and patient, I returned to my suite. I assumed that the good doctor had informed the ship's captain of the attack on Dr. Petrov.

It was now approaching five thirty in the morning. So after a brief description of the situation to Ruth, I turned in for a few more hours of sleep.

In the morning, after breakfast in the suite (I was finished with lemon Danish), I checked on *my patient.* He had had a relatively comfortable night. No fever, the dressings had been changed, and his toes were moving with complete sensation. He was probably over the hump, but in twelve more hours I would be sure.

The lectures went on. The organizers did have to do some rearranging, since Dr. Petrov was scheduled to give his talk today. "Due to illness, his lecture will be postponed." No one flinched, except for Olga seated in the back of the room. All she uttered was a high-pitched, *"Harrumph."* I, apparently, was the only one who took notice.

Today's tour took us to the town of Amalfi on the beautiful southern Italian coast of the same name.

We got off the tender at the town docks, the ship being too big to dock on the shore. First, we took a sightseeing coach along the winding, rocky road to the town of Positano. The city clung to the side of the mountainous coastline. We walked down to the Hotel Sirenuse and had lunch on the veranda looking over the picturesque town as it ran down to the sea. It was inspiring.

Upon returning to Amalfi, we toured the town and even walked up the one hundred steps to the cathedral with its magnificent elevated view of the city and the docks with boats constantly coming and going from such exotic places as the Isle of Capri. Our ship looked small and stately as it rode at anchor in deep water.

Enough touring. We headed down to the docks to board the next tender that was leaving for our ship.

The little boat docked and the sailors expertly tied it down and then launched the boarding platform, which ran between the dock and the tender entrance. I waited until Ruth was safely onboard. The tender was rocking in the choppy sea. I put one foot on the boarding platform and, as I lifted my foot from the dock surface, the boarding plank shifted to my right. With nothing to hold on to, I was thrown off balance to my left. The sailors screamed in Italian and reached for me, but over I went.

You've heard of "hanging on by your fingertips"? Well, that's exactly the situation I found myself in. My feet and lower legs were in the water between the dock and the ship. With the wave action causing the tender to bob and move, my legs were in perfect position to be crushed between the boat and the dock. Fortunately, the sailors on the dock were able to reach me quickly and drag me onto the dock, where I lay panting for a minute or two. Then they helped me to my feet.

The boarding plank was reestablished in a stable position and I was helped aboard the tender by many hands, my shoes squishing with seawater. Ruth was about to have a heart attack. I told her I was fine except for my wet trousers and footwear.

"Did you see what happened?" I asked.

"No, Ham. By the time I turned around to watch you board the tender, you were already in the water."

"Did you see what happened to cause the boarding plank to shift?" I queried.

"No, but there were several men around the plank, on the dock side, and after you fell in one or two of them walked away instead of trying to help you."

"Well, it could have been a lot worse," I said, wringing the seawater out of my trouser legs.

That night, after a good hot shower, Ruth and I sat down with the doctors for dinner. During predinner drinks, we were discussing my dangerous escapade. The Russian sommelier was hovering over the table, serving wine and champagne to the doctors. Suddenly she moved awkwardly to her right and spilled a full glass of red wine down the front of my shirt.

"So sorry, Dr. Marks. You send shirt to laundry. We take good care." And with that she moved off into the dinner crowd.

Everyone at the table was very solicitous as I used a napkin to mop the red wine from my white shirt. All I could think of was, *How did she know my name? There are no nameplates at the table, or on me.* I laughed and said, "This obviously is not my day!"

Ruth and I took in a movie and retired for the night.

"What a day!" Ruth said. "It was almost as if someone was out to get you, Ham."

"Hmmmmm," I said.

As we were preparing to go to bed, but before we had removed our clothes, the little doorbell on our suite door rang. I opened the door, and there standing in his resplendent whites was the ship's captain. A seaman was by his side.

"I know it's late, Dr. Marks, but may we come in for a moment?"

"Why of course, Captain. Come in, come in," I said.

The captain entered, holding his hat in one hand and a white envelope in the other. I, assuming that the envelope was something like an invitation to the captain's table, said, half jokingly, "You didn't have to deliver that personally, Captain."

"What? Oh, no. I found this envelope stuck in your door mail slot. But you certainly will be invited to my table later in the cruise. No, I came to apologize for what happened to you today—both incidents. The terrifying accident you had on the shore, boarding the tender, and the spilling of wine on you during dinner tonight. Both incidents are unforgivable and I offer my deepest apologies, along with the apologies of the ship's owners. In addition, I want you to take this card and replace the clothing items that were ruined today at the ship's stores. The bill will be paid through my account."

With that, he handed me an embossed card that stated, "All items selected by Dr. H. Marks will be charged to the account of Captain Mathew Gillespie."

"Just give the card to any salesperson and take it back if you can't replace everything in one store."

"Why thank you, Captain. I will do that. I ruined a pair of slacks and a good pair of shoes during that ocean swim I inadvertently took, and you know about my shirt with the wine stain."

"Yes, Doctor. Please turn those items over to the seaman here, and we will do our best to revitalize them. But do replace them anyway."

Ruth turned over the slacks, shoes, and shirt to the seaman, and then he and the captain left the suite.

"Well, that was considerate of them," I said to Ruth.

To which she remarked, "And what is the letter all about?"

"Oh, it's probably an invitation to some ship's activity," I said as I opened the envelope addressed to "Dr. Ham Marks."

On a piece of ship's stationery was written in block letters, "STAY AWAY FROM THE DOC. OR IT MIGHT NOT BE WIEN ON SHIRT NEXT TIME."

No signature.

"What the . . . !"

"What does that mean, Ham? Is it a threat?"

"Well, if it is, it's written by someone who took English as a second language in school."

"Don't joke, Ham. Is this about helping that injured doctor the other night?"

"I don't know, dear. But that's over and done with. So let's not let this illiterate note spoil our "C" change, love."

I threw the note in the waste receptacle in the suite. But later on I retrieved it and put it in my attaché case—just in case it might be of some forensic value later on.

We went to bed and, after turning and wrestling with the covers, and visions of other than "sugar plums" in our heads, we fell asleep.

Chapter 7
Qui Bono?

What good is it

A day off—great! I felt like a kid playing hooky. No lectures today.

Ruth and I prepared to visit Sicily. We were landing in Messina and then taking a bus trip to Taormina.

But first we had to avoid Scylla and Charybdis! According to ancient legend, these two death traps for sailors rested between the boot of Italy and the toe of Sicily in the Straits of Messina.

Scylla was a giant nymph rooted to a rocky prominence. She had fierce dog heads around her waist. If sailors came too close, she would reach out and grab them with clawed fingers and feed them to the dogs.

Not too far away was Charybdis, a gaping mouth that was a fearsome whirlpool that would swallow sailors who, in order to avoid Scylla, would sail right into the maelstrom.

The English phrase that described this perilous situation was, "Between a rock and a hard place."

Hopefully, the captain had marked these twin terrors on his GPS and would easily avoid them.

After tying up the *Europa Star*, the crew let us off to stroll around the beautiful Messina port gardens. We then boarded our tourist bus and took the forty-five minute trip to Taormina. This elevated town is a unique blend of the ancient and not so ancient.

At one end of town was the ancient Roman amphitheater that peered down on the Gulf of the Cyclops, named for the one-eyed beast who scared the hell out of Odysseus and his sailors. At the other end of the main street was the Santa Dominica monastery, which was once a religious retreat, then the headquarters of Hitler's SS troops in Sicily, and finally a magnificent, first-class, tourist hotel with gardens overlooking the rocky cliffs that reached down to the sea.

After a tasty lunch in one of Taormina's open-air restaurants, we reboarded the bus and returned to the port. Before reboarding the ship, Ruth's and my attention was drawn to a small crowd of shipboard companions who were standing in a semicircle surrounding a group of men who struck us as dangerous. In the middle of the group was a man dressed like a sheikh: white robes and a head cover held in place by a colorful headband. That was interesting enough, but surrounding the "sheikh" were six men in black suits, all carrying automatic weapons. They looked like AK47s—but then what do I know about AK47s?

"Are they AK47s?" I asked a uniformed ship's officer standing at *Europa's* gangway.

"Yes, sir, they are," he answered unhesitatingly.

"Well, are you planning to allow that group onboard?" I persisted, hoping the officer would understand my concern.

"Oh, yes. That's Sheikh Ahmed el Faisal from Abu Dhabi and his bodyguards. They often join us midcruise. You will hardly notice them onboard. They tend to stay in their suites."

"Well, we certainly hope so," I said, turning to Ruth. "We really don't like being around men brandishing automatic weapons."

"Don't worry, sir. They have never used those weapons yet, and I don't expect them to do so on this trip." The officer's words were reassuring.

Ruth and I entered the ship and rode up in the elevator with fellow shipmates who couldn't stop talking about the sheikh and his men. Ruth and I looked at each other but kept mum. These folks were going to have to register their fears with the ship's crew and get their share of comfort from them—not from us.

We relaxed in our suite and prepared for dinner. I checked the computer for e-mail and Ruth put in a call to her "animal man."

Dinner was excellent. We discussed the day's tourism with our tablemates and my shirt remained spotless, even though I had two glasses of an excellent red wine—served by a new Canadian sommelier.

Ruth and I decided to try our hands (or feet) at dancing after dinner. So we walked to the forward ballroom where a ten-piece band was entertaining the cruisers with oldies but goodies that one could actually dance to without having to be a member of Cirque du Soleil.

We were humming to each other while we tripped the light fantastic, when suddenly our terpsichore came to an abrupt and violent end.

A large body came very close to us and then struck me so hard that both Ruth and I fell to the hardwood floor. Knowing that it would take a hell of a force to knock all 230 pounds of me down, I was concerned with the effects of the blow and fall on Ruth's much lighter body. She said she was all right, and by the time I got her and myself up off the dance floor and looked around, no large body was in sight. I asked a fellow dance couple if they had seen what happened, but they too were swept away by younger memories on the dance floor and could only say that they saw us "on the floor."

Ruth and I retired and applied butler-obtained icepacks to our bruise spots. Ultimately, with the help of a few Tylenol apiece, we fell asleep.

Until three a.m.! The phone rang. I automatically picked it up and said, "Dr. Marks."

A voice answered that I recognized immediately. "Dr. Marks, I'm so sorry."

"Dr. Rosenbaum, what's up?"

"I'm afraid our problem patient has been injured again. This time it's his elbow, and I'm afraid I need your professional help again. The elbow looks like it is dislocated, but I'm getting an X-ray as we speak."

"Okay, Doc. I'll be down in a few minutes. Just pack the elbow in ice and keep a check on his radial pulse."

I explained the situation to Ruth, who by now was wide-awake.

"Ham, what on earth is going on?"

"I don't know, dear, but it looks like Dr. Petrov needs my services again. I'll call you from the infirmary."

Upon entering the stainless steel chamber, once again I was presented with Dr. Petrov in severe pain. He obviously had a dislocated right elbow.

After checking his radial pulse and finding it intact, I turned to Dr. Rosenbaum and said, "Here's what I'm going to need. First, give Dr. Petrov an IV dose of twenty milligrams of Valium. Second, prepare a two-foot plaster splint of three-inch plaster and find me a four-inch Ace bandage. And third, give him an intramuscular injection of Demerol right now."

"Right," said Dr. Rosenbaum as he departed to put together my requirements.

I turned to the patient and said, "Dr. Petrov, how did this happen?"

"Oh, Dr. Marks, it's so good to see you again. I walking on deck again and I saw a big body quickly come up to me, force me into railing, and throw me over rail. I grab top rail with my right hand and stop from going overboard. But pain in elbow awful, and if passing passenger not pull me up, I would be with fishes now."

"Well, I'm glad you're not with the fishes." (I too used the Mafia line for people being drowned in the ocean by bad men.) "We'll have you fixed up in a few moments. But I certainly would suggest that you never again walk on the deck at night by yourself."

"That sound like good advice, Dr. Marks."

After the Demerol and Valium were injected, Dr. Petrov was relaxed and somnolent. I placed Dr. Rosenbaum's hands in position above the patient's elbow to apply countertraction. I then placed gentle but firm traction on Dr. Petrov's hand, in the line of the elbow's deformed position, until a soft *clunk* indicated that the elbow was relocated. I placed the posterior splint, held on with the Ace bandage, between his right upper arm and his hand, in a flexed or bent position at the elbow.

I turned to Dr. Rosenbaum and said, "After a check X-ray, you should have your nurses apply ice packs to the elbow and check the radial pulse hourly for the next eight hours. After that, he should be all right on his own, wearing a sling."

"Fine, I'll take care of that right away. Thank you so much for helping out here."

"No problem," I said.

And then to Dr. Petrov I said, "I'll check on you in the morning, Doctor. You will have to wear the splint for about three weeks and the sling for an additional three weeks, but that shouldn't stop you from doing your normal activities, except perhaps feeding yourself with your right hand until you remove the splint. Okay?"

"Ochaa. Sank you sa much," the medicated doctor slurred.

"You are very welcome, Doctor."

I turned to leave the infirmary and said to Dr. Rosenbaum, "You know how to get a hold of me if you need me, Doc."

"I certainly do. And thank you again, Dr. Marks."

Ruth, of course, was wide-awake and awaiting my tale. After a brief explanation of the situation, and an apology for not calling, we both returned to our state of deep sleep easily.

CHAPTER 8

ALTER EGO

The other person

"You seem very interested in Dr. Petrov's Vanishe cream. Are you a dermatologist?" I asked the big doctor.

The small fellow with the bald spot on the top of his head must have noticed that I had checked on Dr. Petrov's elbow condition during a lecture break.

"No, no, no. I'm an orthopedic surgeon," I said to him.

"Well, it certainly looks like Dr. Petrov could use one of those. I'm Simeone Markov, a pharmacologist from Cleveland. (This is my opportunity to get to know this big fellow who is hanging around the Bulgarian doctor with the valuable new product.)

"I'm Ham Marks from Philadelphia," I said, flashing my badge and extending my hand.

"Oh, Philadelphia. I've been there. Very friendly people," I said while taking his giant mitt in my comparatively rather small hand.

"City of Brotherly Love," I said.

"Is that so? Well, Dr. Marks, how come an orthopedic surgeon from Philadelphia is so interested in a dermatologist from Bulgaria?"

"Bulgaria? I didn't realize that. I just thought it was an interesting product, particularly after I heard Dr. Petrov's lecture."

"A Bulgarian doctor who licenses his product to a Greek company. Interesting, huh?" I queried him again.

"I don't know anything about that," I said.

He looks and sounds innocent enough. But he's got himself mixed up in a bad situation: fixing up Petrov's leg and his elbow. Look what happened to him at the dinner table and on the dance floor. Not to mention the slip *on the gangway in Amalfi. I do keep tabs on folks I'm interested in.*

I also have my eye on those two big thugs from Sofia: Bohdan Ivanchuk and Andrij Babich. They both have records as long as their arms and legs—mostly for muscle stuff, beating up people. They've never killed anybody as far as my people can determine, but they obviously will do anything for money. I'm sure they have something to do with both Dr. Petrov's and Dr. Marks's mishaps. They certainly are pretty sneaky and fast for big men. I don't want to engage them directly in conversation because I don't want them to be aware of my presence.

The Ukrainian doctor from UCLA seems to be just what he says he is and has nothing to do with the trouble.

I can't get a handle on the Belorussian. He keeps slipping in and out of the scene, but I'll tag him sooner or later.

The ship's engineer likes to drink scotch, but he appears also to be outside of the trouble.

The Russian lady intrigues me. I think I'll tackle her next. I'll let her work some of her wiles on me.

I walked away from Dr. Marks.

CHAPTER 9
FIAT LUX

Let there be light

"That's an interesting-looking drink. What's it called?" I asked as I sat down next to the blonde Russian lady.

"It is a flying grasshopper. It has crème de menthe, crème de cacao, and wadka."

"Wadka?"

"Yes, wadka, wadka! You know, Russians drink wadka!"

"Oh, vodka." Like I didn't know.

"Yes, I am Russian, so I drink wadka. What do you drink?"

"Well, my name is Simeone Markov, and I drink light beer. Waiter!"

"Markov is Russian name, no?"

"Well, I grew up in Bulgaria, but now I'm from Cleveland, Ohio."

"Ohio, that is American, no?"

"Yes. I'm a pharmacist here for the cruise medical lecture series. I've seen you there. Are you a doctor?" I asked.

"No, but my father does own a pharmaceutical company, so I go to lectures to learn for him. I am from St. Petersburg. My name is Olga Alexandrova."

"Oh, I see. Then you take the information back to him in St. Petersburg?"

"Yes."

"He's not here with you, is he?"

"Who?"

"Your father."

"No, no, no. He is in St. Petersburg. I am here—alone. Why don't you come to my cabin? I show you pictures of my father's pharmaceutical company, and information about the products he makes."

"Well, I don't know . . ."

"Yes, you come. I have light beer in refrigerator."

"Okay. Just one light beer."

"Yes. Just one."

With that, she slid off the bar stool, grabbed my arm, and just about frog-marched me to her cabin, which was one of the larger suites on the ship. About five times the size of my cabin.

She sat me down at a round dining table and brought over a large, leather-bound photo album, which she placed in front of me.

She then went to the bar refrigerator, opened the door, and bent over to peer inside, giving me a direct view of her long, suntanned legs that led upward to reveal her skimpy white underwear that was barely covered by her short skirt. After enough time to give me an appreciative look, she straightened up with a bottle of light beer in her hand. She brought the beer and a glass to the table and poured the beer expertly.

"Aren't you having anything?" I asked.

"Oh, yes. I make drink for myself soon. But first, I want to show you pictures."

With that, she reached across me and opened the album. At that point, her breasts were resting right on my bald spot. What an interesting sensation!

"You see. It a big company."

She revealed the picture of a large stone structure, about a block long, that was reminiscent of the Hermitage's architecture. On the top of the building was a large sign in Cyrillic, which she translated as "St. Petersburg Pharmaceutical Company." She added, "Big Pharma."

"Nice building," I said.

She jiggled her breasts on my head and turned the page.

"Here some of the products my father makes." She showed me pictures of pharmaceutical bottles with labels that included descriptions of the products, their uses, dosages, and side effects—all in Russian. Perhaps she was testing me. But then she went on (and continued jiggling).

"This one is powerful antibiotic," she said. "This one is anti-AIDS pill. This one cures multiple sclerosis."

All, it would appear, stolen from other countries rather than developed by the "St. Petersburg Pharmaceutical Company."

Then she squatted down next to me, placing her well-manicured hand on my thigh, and began casually rubbing up and down—coming very close to my groin.

"You stay and read and drink beer. I have to change to workout clothes, then I come back and we talk more."

With that, she pressed harder on my upper thigh and stood up. Then she turned and walked into the bedroom portion of the suite, taking her blouse off before she disappeared behind the separation barrier.

At that point, I had a decision to make. I had already gathered significant information. She was, in fact, gathering information for her father, the general. Whether or not she was *alone* was another question. I'll have to answer that for myself at a later time.

The decision having been made, reluctantly, I tiptoed out of the suite and softly closed the door.

CHAPTER **10**

CUM MALEM

With malice

Next stop, Dubrovnik, Croatia (formerly Yugoslavia). The famous red-walled city came into view as the ship approached the central marina and was skillfully docked and tied down.

Ruth and I were eagerly anticipating our visit to this interesting and picturesque city. We exited the shuttle bus and walked slowly toward the city entrance through an arch in the wall.

We were excited to see how a modern population lived inside these ancient, thick red walls. Actually, we were somewhat disappointed when we got inside. It was just like every other touristy European city in which the shop owners attempted to rip you off the best they could.

We walked through a museum, built into the stone wall, to see the history of Dubrovnik. We walked down the cobblestone streets, observing the pockmarks in several of the building sides, made by bullets fired during an old Balkan war.

We sat at an outside table in the city's central square, listening to a small musical group and drinking the local light beer.

We then began slowly strolling back toward the entrance to the walled city and our shuttle bus. We were talking to each other about the unique yet mundane aspects of the city, when we heard a shout. "Look out! Look out! Above you! Above you!"

We suddenly realized that they were pointing and shouting at us!

Rumble, rumble, rumble. I looked up toward this noise, and to my amazement I saw a large red boulder rolling to the edge of the top of the wall. And then falling down, down, down—directly toward Ruth and me.

The road we were on was narrow and there wasn't much room or time to move away from the descending rock.

I pushed Ruth up against the glass window of a store selling overpriced coral jewelry and covered her body with my own. The giant rock fell directly toward us and at the last second struck the steel frame of the awning over the store window. It dropped at our feet.

The sound of the stone striking the ground was like an explosion. I was faced away from the collision, so I didn't see the missile break into dozens of pieces of rock shrapnel, but I did feel several of the pieces strike me in the back. I thought for sure that I had suffered an open wound, but when I reached back I felt no blood and not even a tear in my windbreaker. As luck would have it, the rock fragments had struck my camera case and bounced harmlessly into the street.

Ignoring the jabbering crowd that gathered around us, I said to Ruth, "Are you all right?"

"Yes, and you?"

"I'm fine. Pieces of rock struck my camera case but didn't cut me."

"What was that?" Ruth gasped.

"I don't know. Let's ask someone in the crowd."

"A big rock came off the wall. I think someone pushed it," an English-speaking bystander said.

A policeman hurried up to us and said, in surprisingly good English, "Are you okay, sir?"

"Yes, yes," I said. "But you had better investigate how that rock came down. Either there's something loose up on the wall or someone was trying to harm us."

"Yes, I will investigate. You will please give me your name and your ship, and cabin number, and I will call you."

I did as he asked, thanked him, and escorted Ruth, who was now shaking, quickly out of the gate and onto the bus.

After a drink or two and some hors d'oeuvres served by our butler in our suite, the phone rang. I answered. "Hello. Yes, Officer. Oh, is that right? Well, if anything else turns up, please call the ship, will you? Thank you, Officer."

"Well?" queried Ruth.

"Well," I answered, "the officer found some broken stone on the top of the wall. But he said that it couldn't have fallen by itself."

"Is that good or bad news?"

"It's good news, as long as we're here, drinking booze—in one piece," I said.

CHAPTER 11
ID EST

That is

The ship was moving slowly down the Grand Canal, approaching the marina dock in Venice. The doctors had been given the morning off to watch the approach to Venice.

Ruth had drunk her juice and gone off to her workout class. I slept late, showered, and was sitting down to a sumptuous breakfast of eggs, bacon, coffee, and brioche served by our butler. This doesn't happen in Philadelphia!

I opened the ship's copy of the *Herald Tribune* and was catching up on the sports scores when Ruth reentered the suite with a towel wrapped around her neck.

"I think I'll have my breakfast before I shower. That treadmill workout made me hungry," Ruth said.

"Fine with me, dear. Dig in. It looks delicious."

We both ate in relative silence as I read the paper and Ruth chewed and thought. When Ruth finished and rose to go to the shower, I said, "Put on some comfortable shoes, dear, and we'll take a spin around the deck when you're ready."

"Okay," she said, and then she disappeared into the bathroom.

I finished the paper at the same time that Ruth reappeared, dressed in a sleeveless pink shirt, white shorts, and pink walking shoes. I was wearing khaki Bermuda shorts, a polo shirt, and sneakers.

We left the suite hand in hand and walked out to the deck. This was nice. We hadn't had a chance to walk and talk since we arrived on the *Europa Star*.

Various cruisers jogged by us as we walked. After about five minutes in this mode, I turned to Ruth, and she turned toward me.

"What do you think is going on?" we both said at the same time.

"You first, my dear," I said.

"Ham, what is happening to us? There is either a concerted effort to harm us on the part of some unknown party or we are having a run of the world's worst luck."

"I know, I know," I said. "I can't figure it out either."

"Maybe it has to do with that Dr. Petrov you keep having to take care of, and who is having luck as bad as ours."

"Well, Dr. Rosenbaum has been treating Petrov, and he hasn't been harmed, as far as I know. But then, he isn't a part of the medical conference," I reasoned.

"Who can we talk to about this?" Ruth queried.

"I don't know, dear. The captain knows, and the ship's security officer knows. I'll talk to the doctor who is running the conference, but I don't know what good that will do."

At that moment, two very large men jogged toward us on the deck. Their arms were covered with tattoos. We both stared at them as they approached. When they were about three feet away, they both gave sinister smiles, and one of the giants formed his right hand into the shape of a pistol: thumb up and index finger pointed at us. As they passed, Ruth and I heard them both laughing.

"What was that about?" Ruth said with some trepidation.

"I don't know, dear. But I have a feeling that those two are a part of the problem that we are having."

"Well, what should we do about it?"

"I'll speak to the security officer. Maybe he can have them watched," I said.

"Ham, Why don't you call that nice FBI lady and talk to her," Ruth suggested.

"You mean Linda Carter?"

"Yes."

"Well, I don't know how she could help us, since we're five thousand miles away, but if we have any more *bad luck* I will do just that. I have her number in my iPhone."

"Good!"

We finished our walk uneventfully and went into the dining room for a light lunch.

CHAPTER 12
QUID PRO QUO

This for that

I was walking down the hallway from my room, just walking and thinking. I had to get away from all of those bios pasted on my walls. My thoughts were focused on the Bulgarian doctor, Petrov, and his misfortunes. I had spoken to him about his injuries, but he seemed reticent to talk to me about them—claimed they were accidental. I did get him to open up somewhat about Olympias, the Greek firm to which he had licensed his product. His lecture during the course had been about the European patent and licensing procedures. So he was agreeable to talking to me, at his booth, about his experience.

He told me that the Greeks had offered the best terms for royalties of all the companies he had approached. I asked him why he didn't go with a Ukrainian or Russian company that would be undoubtedly bigger than the Greek company.

He made a terrible face, as if he had just swallowed a jalapeno pepper and was about to spit it out. But what came out of his mouth was, "They are Mafia! And I do not do business with Mafia!"

I smiled to myself, and just then I saw the two Ukrainian thugs approaching me with ugly smiles on their faces. Frick went to my left, Frack went right, and I was left staring straight ahead into the empty hallway. Suddenly one thug shoved his arm under one armpit while the other grabbed my opposite side. They picked me up off the carpeted floor and began carrying me backward down the hallway.

I was so shocked that for a moment I couldn't say anything. Then I regained my composure and began to shout. "What are you doing? Put me down! You can't do this to me!"

While I was shouting, I was thinking. (I'm a multitasker.) I know these two bozos, but they don't know who I am—or I least who I really am. And since I didn't have my weapon handy, there wasn't much sense in telling them. Then I thought of a saying taught to me by one of my Case Western classmates as we were both waiting to go in for our oral exams: "We also serve who only stand and wait." So I shut up.

The two heavyweights reached the end of the corridor. They opened a cabin door, threw me in, and locked the door. Just then I learned something. You can lock a cabin door from the outside.

Having failed to open the door, no matter how hard I twisted or pulled on the knob, I gave up and looked around the cabin. I knew this place! Just as I got my head on straight and began to figure out exactly where I was, in walked Olga, all of her—in the buff! Or almost in the buff. She had on a G-string that almost covered her pubic area—but not quite. Her abundant pubic hair overflowed the little patch. Her voluptuous breasts were completely uncovered. No nipple tassels, no nothing!

Now I have seen topless ladies on Ukrainian beaches before, but this was well beyond that. All she had on were her red high-heeled pumps.

"You left too soon last time, Meester Simeone Markov. Now I haf you all to myself."

With that, she took both of my shoulders in her hands and literally threw me down on the couch. She leaped on top of me, wriggling like a snake with hiccups. With one motion, she unzipped my fly and started massaging my semierect member.

"Wait!" I said.

She stopped wriggling and massaging.

"What? You vant a light beer first, then we fuck?" she said nonchalantly.

"Yes," I said firmly.

"Okay. Ve drink—then we fuck," she said, getting up and going to bend over at her icebox, giving me a much less impeded bodily view than I had had the last time.

She brought the bottle of light beer, top removed, to me and poured a large vodka over ice for herself.

She sat on the couch and leaned back with her legs spread.

"Vat you vant to talk about vile ve drink?" she asked.

"I want to know what you want in return," I said.

"In return for vat?"

"You know, in return for your *favors*," I answered.

"My favors? Oh, my favors! Vell, now dat you ask, I tell you."

"Yes, please do," I encouraged, trying to relax with the cold beer in my hand.

"Vell, I vould like you to find out something for me."

"Okay. What's that?"

"I vant you to find out vat kind of deal Petrov has vith the Greek company for his Wanishe cream."

"Well, you already know that he licensed his patent to them for royalties."

"Da, da, but did he assign the patent to them? How long is the agreement for?"

"You want me to find out all that for your *favors?*"

"Yes. You tink you can do it?"

"I'll certainly give it a try," I said, trying not to upset her plan.

"Dat's good," she said. "Now ve fuck."

With that, she whipped off her G-string and pounced on me once again.

"Wait!" I said. This was getting difficult.

"Vat now?" she said, sitting down with her legs spread across my midsection.

"This is not fair."

"Fair?" she said.

"Yes," I said. "I haven't paid off yet. Why don't I get the information first, come back and give it to you, and then you give me *your favors.*"

"Okay. Dat's a good deal. I let you out; you get information and come back and we fuck. I vait like dis."

"Well, it might take some time," I said. "Why don't you get dressed and wait for my call?"

"Vell . . . Okay."

And with that, she jumped off of me and went to the door—stark naked. She took a room key out of a desk drawer and opened the door wide for me. "You hurry back," she said. "I very horny for you."

I hurried out the door, zipping my fly, and she slapped me on my backside before closing the door.

The giant thugs were nowhere in sight as I turned down the corridor.

Well, I thought, *at least I know what she's after. And I also know that I will need my holstered weapon on my person from now on.*

CHAPTER 13

VENEZIA

Venice

The *Europa Star* docked at the Venice marina dock around noon. Ruth and I had a lovely lunch in the ship's dining room and then prepared, in our suite, to go out sightseeing until dinnertime.

We left the ship and after a short walk came to the nearby water taxi station, marked by a red-and-white-striped pole that looked like a barber's. We bought tickets to St. Mark's Square and then had a foreigner's good time figuring out which boat would take us where we wanted to go.

Fortunately, we chose correctly. After cruising down the Grand Canal for a time, stopping at intermediate stops along the way, we departed the watercraft at St. Mark's Square.

We walked along stones into the center of the square with hundreds of pigeons walking around us and flying over us. Ruth was fascinated. I was trying to recall my first-year med school course on infectious diseases to determine how long it would take, if I inhaled any of these wafting pigeon feathers, to develop psittacosis (a lung disease carried on bird feathers). That thought temporarily dampened my ardor at being here in Venice. But soon I had my camera out and was snapping the same pictures that adorned all of the packages of postcards for sale at the souvenir kiosks.

We passed the magnificent St. Mark's Cathedral, the Doge's Palace, the Bell Tower, and, of course, the towering obelisk erected to Saint Mark.

Ruth took her own pictures, so now we had two sets of postcard scenes.

We continued walking and passed under an arch in the stone that surrounded the square. We found ourselves on an ancient street between small stores and restaurants. At the end of the street, we strolled over one of the arched bridges crossing the small canals running through Venice instead of streets. No car traffic, only small motorboats and gondolas.

At the end of the bridge was a building whose entrance was overarched by a sign that said, in golden letters, "Venezia Antica. Venetian Glassworks." We entered and were immediately overwhelmed. Everything was made of magnificent colored glass. There were horses, large birds, Chinese figures, and candelabras of all sizes. We were turning in circles with wonder. We then went deeper into the building and watched a demonstration of glass blowing. Ruth and I left the building agreeing that we would have to come back when we had more time to buy a piece for our home.

We joined a group of doctors from our ship for tea and pastries outside of one of the restaurants. During our conversation with our fellow cruisers, we made a date with another doctor and his wife to take a private launch on a ride up the Grand Canal the next day, since we had another full day in Venice tomorrow.

After tea, we returned to the public launch and sailed back to the ship in plenty of time for a nice nap before dinner.

CHAPTER 14
DEATH IN VENICE

I've been to Venice several times, mainly for the service, but I wouldn't mind having a coffee in St. Mark's Square and people watching. It would be a fun challenge for me to sit there and try and pick out the "bad" guys.

As I contemplated a lazy day, my cabin phone rang.

"Emergency, emergency, sir. This is the first officer calling for the ship's captain. Please meet us in cabin 303, the cabin of Olga Alexandrova, right away. There has been a critical accident."

"I'll be right there," I said, thinking, *Critical accident?* That's a code for a death. I immediately left my cabin, but not before checking my weapon and placing it in my shoulder holster under my light jacket.

Olga's cabin was just down the long corridor from mine and was unforgettable, as far as I was concerned.

I arrived to find the captain, the first officer, and the doctor just inside the open cabin door. There was also another man. After a short stare, I recognized him from my wall pictures as the Ukrainian doctor from UCLA who had given the abstruse lecture on AIDS care.

This time I was introduced as a representative from the Bulgarian Secret Service. I shook hands with the doctor and then extended my hand to the other "doctor" in the room. The questioning look on my face said, "Who the hell are you?"

It was my fault. I hadn't gotten a good handle on this one. And so I was surprised, if not floored, when the captain said to me, "Simeone, Frank Sturgis here is a representative of the US Intelligence Service."

116

"Oh," I said. "The CIA, for heaven's sake. What are they doing here? And what a great disguise. It actually fooled me—temporarily."

"Yes, Simeone, we had good info that there might be some international illegal drug deals going on here, and that's where I come in," Sturgis said.

I was embarrassed that I had been fooled, so I turned away from the CIA man. Immediately a sour, metallic smell struck me: blood, and lots of it, on the cabin floor, along with the naked, and obviously dead body of Olga Alexandrova. With one red shoe on and the other lying far across the room.

The doctor was kneeling down and examining the body.

"Blunt trauma to the head," he said, placing his gloved hand into a large, bloody wound at the back of Olga's skull.

I looked around and found blood on the sharp corner of the coffee table in front of the couch from which I had negotiated my way out of her amorous clutches.

"Looks like she fell—or was pushed—and struck her head on the sharp point of this table," I said.

"Why was she naked?" the CIA man asked. He knew who she was and who she represented.

All present were silent, but I knew the answer to the query. She was trying to entice some poor man into doing something she wanted him to do, and was repulsed violently.

"Doctor," the captain said, "is this an accidental death or a homicide?"

"I don't know for sure, Captain. But from the depth of the wound in her skull, I would lean toward her being thrown against the table. In that case, there is probably another person involved in her death."

I agreed with that evaluation. I checked the couch and removed the cushions. There were several coins, along with two champagne corks and cocktail napkins.

The coins consisted of two US quarters, one US dime, one Canadian quarter, and one gold coin, the size of a US quarter, with "25" on it and the portrait of a man in modern dress with "Alexander" over his head. "Lukashenko" was below his torso. I knew where this latter coin came from: Belarus. I knew of only one Belorussian on this cruise: the doctor on the medical conference list, Victor Archovy, whom I had crossed off my list as "no trouble." Could I be wrong twice?

I turned the coins over to the captain but kept my supposition as to where the coin covered with the face of the elected dictator of Belarus had come from.

Just then, I realized that there was one man missing from the assembled group. Where was the ship's security officer? Surely he should be here collecting evidence and preparing for an arrest—or at least preparing a list of passengers to question.

The captain's cell phone rang.

"Yes, Arthur. Okay, I will leave the doctor and the first officer here and meet you in the cabin shortly. Thank you."

"That was my security officer, Arthur Root," the captain explained, putting his cell phone away. "He was called to investigate a commotion, a man screaming in cabin 506. He's there now, and the occupant of the cabin is also there—having been badly beaten."

I knew who occupied cabin 506. His face was on the wall of my cabin. It was the Belarusian doctor, Victor Archovy. I must be slipping.

The captain, the CIA officer, and I went down the corridor and took the elevator to the fifth floor. We entered cabin 506 and found Root talking with a man in obvious distress. I knew it was Victor Archovy, but he certainly didn't look like the picture on my cabin wall.

Both of Archovy's eyes had been blackened. He was holding an ice bag to his obviously bruised jaw, and he was holding the right side of his chest and having difficulty breathing, because of what I assumed to be multiple rib fractures.

I stood by while the captain took out his phone and struck a speed-dial number. "Doctor, I think you had better get to room 506 as soon as possible. The man in the cabin is injured and needs your attention immediately. Thank you, Doctor."

The security officer was still talking softly to Victor Archovy. He was mainly calming the man, who was almost in shock.

I kept quiet and listened. The captain asked the security chief to explain what had happened. At that moment, the doctor arrived and attended to Dr. Archovy.

The security chief spoke to the captain in my presence and in front of the CIA fellow. "Dr. Archovy is from Belarus. He doesn't know anyone aboard, except for the doctors he has met during this cruise. He was returning to his cabin this afternoon. He had turned the key in his door when he was violently shoved into his cabin. Then two large men beat and kicked him for about ten minutes. They left him lying on his cabin floor. He can't identify his attackers, and he has no idea why they beat him. He feels it's a case of mistaken identity."

"Captain," I said, "I was also attacked, but not beaten, by two large men. I can point them out to you, if you wish. They are known thugs from Sofia, Bulgaria, and I think they work for the dead lady, Olga Alexandrova. Take a look at one of the coins I gave you. It's Belarusian. Unless you can recall having other Belarusian citizens on your ship, I would have to assume that the coin came from the pocket of Dr. Archovy."

"But what was he doing in her cabin?" the captain asked.

"I don't know," I said, "but first things first. Let's prove that he was actually there—and then confront him with the evidence."

The CIA man spoke up. "I have a fingerprinting kit in my bag. What if I take his prints, saying it was part of the investigation of his being attacked. Then I'll try and match his prints with prints I pick up from the dead lady's room."

"Sounds like a good plan," the captain said.

The security officer and I agreed.

CHAPTER 15
CITY OF CANALS

Back on the *Europa Star*, after our short visit to Venice, Ruth and I noticed an air of excitement. Something had happened in our absence. I asked one of the ship's officers as we entered the dining room. All he would say was, "I don't know anything about that, sir."

The dinner was superb. Just what I needed: another superb dinner!

As Ruth and I meandered back to our own stateroom to watch a Blu-ray movie, Ruth suggested, "Why don't you call your friend Dr. Rosenbaum? He's actually a senior officer on the ship. If anything of import is going on, he probably will know something about it."

"Good idea, dear," I agreed.

As soon as we got comfortable in front of our fifty-inch, flat-screen TV, I picked up the house phone and dialed the doctor's number.

"Hello, this is Dr. Rosenbaum."

"Doctor, it's Ham Marks."

"Oh, Ham, how are you? Our favorite patient, Dr. Petrov, appears to be doing well."

"That's good, Doc. Is anything else going on involving the health of participants in the medical course?"

"As a matter of fact, there were two serious medical incidents, one involving a doctor at the conference, Dr. Archovy from Belarus. The other was an interested bystander at the lecture series, Olga Alexandrova from Russia."

"What happened? I'm all ears."

"Ham, since you are a medical consultant, I will trust you with this information, but you must keep it to yourself. Is that okay?"

"That's fine. Who would I tell anyway?"

"Well, the Belarusian, Dr. Archovy, was beaten severely about the face and body in his cabin. His eyes were blackened. His zygomatic arch and his jaw were fractured, and he has multiple rib fractures."

"My goodness. That sounds like a severe and violent beating," I said.

"Right," said Dr. Rosenbaum. "The second incident was worse. Olga Alexandrova struck her head so severely on a corner of her coffee table that the blow crushed her skull and killed her. She was found naked except for one shoe."

"My goodness!" I exclaimed. "That's awful. Was there any connection between the two events?"

"We don't know, but a Belarusian coin was found on Olga's couch and the security officers onboard are trying to connect the two incidents by finding, if they can, fingerprints of Dr. Archovy in Ms. Alexandrova's cabin."

"Well, let me know what happens, will you, Doc? With all these traumatic events happening to Dr. Petrov, Ruth and me, and now these two, I'm thinking of contacting my FBI friend in Philadelphia. One more bad happening, and I will."

"Please let me know if you do, Ham. And I will notify the security personnel and the captain," Dr. Rosenbaum responded.

"I certainly will. Thank you for trusting me with this information, Doctor."

"You're welcome," Dr. Rosenbaum responded.

With that, I hung up the phone.

"Well?" Ruth questioned.

"Well," I said, "a lot went on while we were off the ship." Then I told her about the two traumatic occurrences.

"That's bad, Ham," Ruth said. "Time to call Lisa Carter?"

"Not quite yet. We'll let the ship's security team work on it for a while. But one more incident and I will call her."

We watched a movie about a soldier going back and back and back into an explosion in a train and finally finding an atomic bomb. It was very scary and looked very real on the big screen, in Blu-ray.

We slept fairly well, considering the bad news we had to digest.

We awoke to a glorious day in Venice. After breakfast in our suite, we called Dr. and Mrs. Brown and arranged to meet them on shore, directly outside the ship's gangway.

There, we reintroduced ourselves to the folks we had met over tea yesterday. "We're Ruth and Ham Marks, from Philadelphia." I said, extending my hand.

"Well, Ham, I'm Roger, and my wife's name is Gloria. We're from Minnesota."

"Okay, Roger, let's go rent a launch for a few hours and enjoy ourselves in the City of Canals."

"Fine," Roger Brown said.

Close by the ship we engaged one of the motorboat launches, all wood and shiny. We expressed ourselves as best we could as to our desire to motor down the Grand Canal and visit the sites. We were not sure how well the boat captain and his crewman understood us, but we understood "$400" clearly. We stepped aboard the sleek motorboat, with the help of the mate, seated ourselves on the leather cushions, and off we went. There was a great deal of boat traffic on the Grand Canal, but outside of some waves gently rocking our boat we motored along without difficulty.

First stop was the Bridge of Sighs. We disembarked the launch and walked across the white limestone-covered arch. The ancient bridge across the Grand Canal allowed us to look up and down the waterway. After seeing the magnificent mansions *floating* on either side, we reboarded the launch and headed to our second stop: the Peggy Guggenheim Museum of Modern Art. The launch let us off on the piazza outside the museum, the gift of an American billionaire family. We spent thirty minutes inside, considering the modern art. It was not really to my taste.

Then back aboard, we headed toward Lido Island across from St. Mark's Square. The vessel traffic remained busy, with larger launches plying the waters up and down the main canal. We saw smaller boats, like ours, and man-operated gondolas scooting in and out of the smaller canals entering the main waterway. We were chatting, smiling, and luxuriating in the cool air as we moved along.

Suddenly my eye fell on a launch carrying four men and coming out of a side canal. Instead of turning up or down the canal, this launch was heading directly toward us.

"Hey!" I shouted out, thinking that perhaps the driver of the boat couldn't see us right in front of them for some reason. But they didn't stop, or veer off, and now everyone onboard our boat was waving and crying out in warning.

"Stop!"

"Veer off!"

"Don't hit us!"

But on they came, and it became obvious to us all that they were intentionally heading right at us. Finally, our captain took action to avoid collision and veered away, causing our boat to tilt sharply. The other boat came to within ten feet of colliding with us and then also veered off sharply, its passengers laughing uproariously as if it were a big joke. Our boat, already tilted about sixty degrees from the captain's emergency maneuver, was now struck by the generated large wake as the other boat veered off.

Ruth and I held on for dear life to the upside gunwale, thinking for two horrible seconds that we were going to capsize. Dr. and Mrs. Brown didn't have two seconds. Dr. Brown flew violently and struck his head against the lower gunwale. He went down on the deck dazed and bleeding from his head with canal water pouring over him. Mrs. Brown was not even that fortunate. She flew over the side of the launch and into the canal. By some miracle, she was able to hang on to the gunwale with one hand.

"Stop the boat!" Ruth and I screamed at the captain, and he immediately threw the throttles into neutral, righting the boat at a standstill.

I immediately stepped to the opposite side of the launch and grabbed Mrs. Brown by both wrists. As I hauled her into the boat, she was sputtering and spitting up rancid canal water.

Ruth tended to Dr. Brown, who was dazed and obviously concussed but was not bleeding badly. She laid him flat on the deck, with his head on a small cushion.

"Do you have any ice onboard?" she asked the captain.

"*Si, signora*," the captain responded. He said something to a crewman, who wrapped Mrs. Brown's dripping wet body in a dry blanket. The crewman then offered Ruth a bag of ice, which she placed against Dr. Brown's bruised head, and she wrapped him in a blanket.

Ruth and I were soaked from spray and water that had come into the boat, but we were unhurt, thankfully. Sirens began to wail and I thought for a moment that I was back on Spruce Street in Philadelphia. These sirens, however, came from two police launches that roared up and attached themselves to both sides of our craft.

Two armed Italian policemen boarded the boat and immediately questioned our captain.

The senior policeman then turned to us and in broken English said, "I am so sorry this happens to you, ladies and men. This is very rare to happen—two boat colliding. We apologize a lot. But first we must contact your ship and have doctor meet us, as we get you back as quickly as possible."

With that, the policemen helped Dr. and Mrs. Brown onboard the first police launch and immediately took off with sirens screaming and the radioman talking, presumably, to the captain of the *Europa Star*. With slightly less speed, Ruth and I were helped aboard the second police vessel and took off at a similar speed with sirens going full blast.

All I could think of at that moment was, *Thank God Ruth and I are all right, and what a shame it is that the Italian boatman was out his $400.*

CHAPTER 16

SINE DIE

Without one more day

So I miss a lovely day in Venice. Duty first! The CIA guy took several fingerprint samples from Olga's cabin (including mine, since I had explained that I had been there *on business*). He fingerprinted Dr. Archovy and me as well as himself as a control and then sent all the prints via satellite to the FBI lab in Washington, DC. He got the results back this morning. Ain't technology grand!

He had two matches. The first was me—no surprise. But the second was Dr. Victor Archovy. So Archovy had been in Olga's cabin and we had the proof. I offered to confront him with the evidence and try and get a confession from him, since I knew, to a great extent, what he had faced in that cabin.

I knocked on Dr. Archovy's cabin door and announced who I was. When he opened the door, I saw a face that wasn't on my cabin wall. At first glance, he reminded me of a human raccoon—a raccoon with a broken nose.

His eyes were blackened, and he wore an adhesive splint over the bridge of his nose where the doctor had manipulated it back to a more or less straight position. His speech was breathless, since his fractured ribs hurt him like hell every time he took a breath. He wore a rib belt, but that just barely allowed him to breath.

I showed him my credentials and asked if he minded me asking a few questions. I actually had brought along a rolling table with coffee, milk, sugar, cookies, and cakes supplied by the cabin steward.

When he invited me in, I stepped aside, got in back of the table, and pushed it into the cabin, saying, "I thought you might like a little snack. I'll bet you haven't been out of your cabin for a meal since your accident."

He shook his head in the negative and croaked, "Thanks. I appreciate that."

His cabin included a couch, a coffee table, and two chairs, in addition to his bed. I wheeled the table up to the couch and moved one chair on one side, signaling to the doctor to sit down, and I sat in the chair on the opposite side. Before I started with my interrogation, I poured a cup of coffee for him and me and passed him the cookies.

I took a sip of the coffee and said, "You know the fingerprints we took of you yesterday?"

He nodded and said something like, "Uh huh." His jaw, fortunately, had only been bruised badly and not broken. But the swelling made speech and cookie eating somewhat difficult.

"Well," I continued, "we found a match to your fingerprints in Olga Alexandrova's cabin. You know, the Russian lady who was killed by a blow to her skull."

His eyes widened, and he started to dribble coffee down the front of his shirt. I passed him a napkin and said, "They found my fingerprints, as well."

He cocked his head to one side and gave me a questioning look. I then gave him the whole story of my visit with Olga, including her jumping on me in her altogether, and my "deal" to get information from Dr. Petrov in order to get away from her. Then I shut up.

He coughed and winced in pain. He took a deep breath and croaked, "The same thing happened to me. She enticed me into her room to show me pictures of her father's pharmacology company, since my family also owns a drug company in Minsk. My brother runs it.

"Then she suggested that I might like to join her in producing Vanishe cream, Dr. Petrov's product. I didn't know what to say, since I really couldn't understand the intent of her request. Then she left the room for a few moments. She returned completely naked and leaped on top of me, wriggling and reaching for my fly. Now, I am not a prude, or a homosexual, but I looked upon this action of hers as an assault. I reacted instinctively. I pushed her off of me—strongly. She flew off of the couch, backward, and struck her head on the coffee table.

"Blood was coming from her head where she hit the table. I slapped her face and called, 'Olga, Olga! Speak to me!' but she was unconscious. I was scared. So I got up and left the cabin and returned to my room.

"Within minutes, someone knocked on my cabin door. When I asked, 'Who is it?' a man's voice answered, 'The steward.' I opened the door and these two huge men pushed me down and started to beat me. They never said a word and left me lying there on the floor.

"The real steward found me and called security. The rest you know."

He finished and just about passed out from the effort of his retelling of his misadventure.

I let him recover with a few moments of silence. And then I said, "I certainly understand your circumstances. You really didn't know at the time that the blow to Olga's head had killed her, did you?"

"Nooo!" he cried. "I just thought she had knocked herself unconscious. I am so sorry," he sobbed. "And who were those men? Did they work for her?"

"Well, I thought they did," I answered. "But she was dead by the time that they attacked you. Those thugs don't do anything on their own, so their present boss must still be onboard. That's something that ship's security will have to work on. Your problem is that you are involved in a homicide. I understand your position, but I'm afraid that you are going to have to answer to the authorities."

"Yes, I know," he said dejectedly.

"I'll send the security chief in to record the story you told me. Is that all right with you?"

"Oh, yes. What will happen to me then?"

"I suppose," I explained, "the authorities will take you off the ship in Corfu, our final port. Then they'll accompany you back to Belarus and turn you over to the local authorities for a judicial decision. I would hope that your explanation would allow for a merciful decision. I'll press security not to place you in handcuffs, if you would like me to."

"Yes, please. And thank you for your understanding."

I shook the doctor's hand and left his cabin. I had some thinking to do.

I telephoned the security chief and told him that Dr. Archovy was waiting for him to give him his confession. I told him he probably should take a secretary who is a licensed notary to take down the story and attest to it. I also asked him to be "kind" to the doctor after he heard his story.

I walked back to my cabin and made a note on the photos on the wall. Beneath the photo of Olga, I wrote, "Deceased." Under Dr. Archovy,

I wrote, "Confessed to Olga's accidental death." Finally, under the two Bulgarian thugs, Bohdan Ivanchuk and Andrij Babich, I wrote, "May have committed assault and battery. Still at large—but not for long!"

I then sat at my desk and contemplated the situation. It would appear that Olga decided to branch out on her own once she got her hands on Dr. Petrov's patent for Vanishe cream. I'm sure that would have made Papa, the general, very angry. Maybe Papa ordered the attack on Dr. Archovy, once he learned that his daughter was dead. But that would leave Papa's messenger or messengers still unknown. I'd have to work on that angle.

CHAPTER 17
MOB

Man overboard

The action in our cabin reminded me of a funeral wake: everyone eating, and talking, and clucking with sympathy over the dunking of Ruth and me. Fortunately, no one had died.

The Browns were still recovering from their wounds in their cabin. The doctor checked them both out and found Mrs. Brown "wet and wild." Dr. Brown was a different case. He had suffered a scalp laceration and a probable concussion. He did not need sutures in his scalp but would require daily neurologic examinations for the remainder of the trip and a CAT scan of his skull as soon as he got home. A skull X-ray, done onboard, had revealed no fractures.

Ruth was pretty much over the acute anxiety she had suffered after almost being thrown into the Grand Canal from our rental motorboat. We both had soiled clothes, but the captain gave us another crack at his credit card to replace our soaked and contaminated clothes and shoes in various shipboard stores. If this continued, Ruth and I would have an entirely different wardrobe when we got off this ship.

Ruth cornered me in a quiet part of the suite. "Ham, I think it's time to call Linda Carter," she whispered.

"I was thinking the same thing, dear," I responded. "I thought I'd call after dinner. It's a six-hour difference, so if I call at ten p.m., it'll be four p.m. at home."

"Good plan," Ruth said, patting me approvingly on the shoulder.

The room cleared, except for one of the ship's officers who approached us and said, "If there is anything else we can do for you, please let us know."

"Thank you, Officer," I said. "Just make sure that Dr. and Mrs. Brown are okay."

"Oh, you can be sure I will. And will you please join us at the captain's table at seven tonight? We cast off at eight thirty, and we will have to be on the bridge at that time."

"We'll be there. And thank you."

With that, the officer saluted us and exited from our suite.

"Well, quite a day." Ruth sighed.

"I'm still concerned that the motorboat captain didn't get paid."

"Oh, Ham. Stop that!"

"I'm kidding, I'm kidding," I said with a chuckle.

We relaxed a bit with drinks from the bar: wine for Ruth and diet root beer for me. Then we showered and dressed for dinner.

Ruth wore her fanciest silk red dress, with silver high heels, to impress the captain. Dinner was delightful. The Browns joined us. The doctor had a small patch on his head where he had struck the gunwale.

The dinner started off with an *amuse-bouche* (I think it was chopped tomato on raw tuna, on toast). I avoided that. Then veal consommé followed by poached sea scallops with mango chutney. That was followed by *filet de boeuf* with truffled wild rice.

There was a glass of the appropriate wine with each course, and an after-dinner liqueur following the dessert of baked Alaska. Coffee was optional.

I know all this because I stole a menu for Ruth's memoirs.

After this sumptuous dinner, we strolled back to our suite and stood on our veranda to watch our departure from Venice on our way to Corfu, the last stop on our "C" change cruise.

The nighttime visage of Venice disappearing behind us was beautiful.

We came inside at nine o'clock to watch the day's world events on Fox News. I had an hour to wait before calling my FBI gal.

At nine thirty, just when Bill O'Reilly was coming on, the ship began to shudder, and the ship's horn gave out the loudest, longest blast I have ever heard.

"Now what?" cried Ruth, whose eyes were as big as teacups.

"I don't know, dear, but I think we're coming to a stop."

"Stop! We're almost in the middle of the ocean!" Ruth said anxiously.

"I don't think we're in the ocean, but we are a few miles from Venice."

With that nautical guesstimate, a voice came over the loudspeaker in our suite.

"Man overboard! Man overboard! This is the captain speaking. This is not a drill. Please go to your cabin and stay there until the all clear is sounded so that the crew can effect an emergency rescue of a person who has gone overboard. Please, stay in your cabin! Thank you."

At the end of the announcement, the ship gave a long shudder, which actually rattled our teeth as well as all the glassware in the suite. We came to a complete stop and began rocking slowly in the sea swells.

Let's go out on the veranda and see what's going on," I said.

"Shouldn't we stay in the cabin?" Ruth admonished.

"The veranda is part of our cabin, but if you want to stay inside that's all right," I said.

"No, no, no!" Ruth said emphatically. "I go where you go."

And out we went.

The sight was not one a tourist cruiser would ordinarily expect to see. Bright floodlights lit the water for one hundred yards in all directions. Crews were lowering motorized lifeboats. Bullhorns manned by the ship's officers were shouting in several languages. Ruth and I were mesmerized.

Several lifeboats began to move away from the side of the ship, moving in larger and larger arcs until one boat began to blow its air horn repeatedly. The rest of the boats formed a circle around what looked like a body brilliantly lit by all the boats. One boat moved in. The crewmen pulled the body aboard. The man or woman appeared lifeless.

The sex of the overboard person was difficult to determine at first. But then it became obvious that it was a man wearing trousers and a jacket. All Ruth and I could make out in trying to identify the person, who appeared to have drowned in the choppy seawater, was that the man had long white hair.

The boat carrying the body moved to the platform on the side of the *Europa Star* and crewmembers and others helped to move the body into our ship.

"Look, there's the doctor," Ruth said, pointing to a short man in a white uniform with staff officer epaulets.

"And there's that 'little man' you keep talking about."

"Who?" I said.

"The fellow with the bald spot in the back of his head. Look! There!" Ruth pointed over the railing.

"Well, I'll be. You're right. I could tell that bald spot anywhere. I wonder what Simeone Markov, the pharmacologist, is doing down there with the ship's bigwigs. It would appear that he's more than just a pharmacologist from Cleveland, doesn't it?"

"It sure does, Ham. We'll have to ask the doctor about him. They seem to be working together," Ruth observed.

The show was finally over. The bright lights gradually winked out as the lifeboats were brought up to their racks on the *Europa's* deck. Ruth and I came in from our veranda and shut the sliding glass door.

The PA system in the room crackled to life.

"This is the captain speaking. The man overboard exercise is over. The crew has successfully brought the person onto the *Europa Star*." Then came a pause. "We will be returning to our berth in Venice. I will speak to you later about your further transportation. As of now, it does not appear that the *Europa Star* will be traveling on to Corfu. Thank you for your attention. Good night." With that, the ship's horn sounded several short blasts signaling "All clear."

Ruth and I looked at each other and spoke at once. "What will we do about . . ."

We both stopped speaking. I said, "I'm sure, dear, that the ship company will arrange our passage to the United States. We'll probably fly home from Venice. There's a direct USAir flight every day to Philadelphia."

"Okay," Ruth said with halfhearted relief.

And then the phone rang. I picked up the receiver and heard the voice of my frequent late-night caller. "Dr. Marks, this is Dr. Rosenbaum."

"Well, hi, Doc. You've had a busy night."

"Yes, I have. I'm sorry to say that we both know the man who went overboard. It was Dr. Petrov."

"Oh, my goodness," I said. "Is he dead?"

"Yes, I'm afraid so. It looks like a small motorboat ran over him in the water and just about decapitated him."

"Oh, that's awful! The poor man. Do we know how he got in the water?"

"Not for certain," said Dr. Rosenbaum. "But it does look like he was thrown overboard, particularly with the history we both have on his series of 'accidents.'"

"Yes. And if he was thrown overboard, I would sure look to those two foreign giants," I speculated.

"Yes, I did mention them to Simeone."

"Simeone," I said. "Simeone Markov, the pharmacologist from Cleveland with the bald spot on the back of his head?"

"Why yes. Do you know him?"

"He takes the medico-legal course with me," I explained.

"Oh, well he's more than just a pharmacologist," the doctor explained. "He's a member of the Bulgarian Secret Service."

"The Bulgarian Secret Service!" I said loudly enough for Ruth to pop out of the bathroom.

With upturned palms, she said, "What is it? Are you all right?"

"Yes, I'm fine, but I just found out that Simeone Markov is a member of the Bulgarian Secret Service."

"Whaaat?" Ruth mouthed.

I held out my hand, palm down, and listened to the doctor on the phone.

"Yes, and there's also a CIA agent onboard. Apparently they were following up some pretty good leads on a drug deal—or something like that."

"Well, I'll be," I said. "Is there anything I can do for you, Doc?"

"No, thank you. I just thought you ought to know about the fate of your patient."

"Well, thanks for the info. If you need me, just call."

"Thanks, Ham. Good night." He hung up.

It took me quite a while to close my lower jaw, which hung open in a stupefied face.

"I think we ought to call Linda Carter now, don't you, Ham?"

"Yes, dear. I do."

I tapped my phone and entered Linda Carter's name at the Philadelphia FBI offices.

She answered on the second ring. "Special Agent Linda Carter."

"Linda, it's Ham Marks, remember me?"

"Ham, would you believe that I was just sitting here recounting in my mind our shootout at the horse farm. Is that amazing?"

"Amazing, but I've got a new story for you, and this time I'm on a ship docked in Venice, Italy."

"Now that does sound interesting. Tell me everything."

"This is a case that I somehow got myself involved in while on a vacation cruise. It involves murder and drugs."

"Now that's my kind of case. Tell me more."

And I did for the next thirty minutes, ending with the dead body being brought aboard *Europa Star* after having been thrown overboard.

There was silence on the other end of the line.

Then she said, "Ham."

"Yes, Linda."

"Can you stay out of trouble until late tomorrow morning?"

"I think so. Yes."

"The FBI recently instituted a worldwide task force against terrorism and illegal drug trading. I think this case fits right in. I'll attach myself to the task force and jump on a government jet. I'll be in Venice in the morning. How's that sound?"

"That's great. When you come aboard, why don't you speak with the captain and the chief security officer? Also there's a Bulgarian Secret Service man, Simeone Markov, and a CIA man you probably ought to touch base with before you come to see us."

"I'll take your advice, Ham. I'll see you and Ruth tomorrow." She hung up.

I turned to Ruth and said, "She'll be here tomorrow. She asked me to stay out of trouble until then."

"Very good advice."

We sat on the couch holding hands and watched the nightly news. Then, with very little conversation, we got ready for bed and fell into a sound sleep.

CHAPTER 18

MENS SANA IN CORPORA SANO

Sound of mind and body

I must be slipping. But I'll deny it if anyone asks.

Olga Alexandrova must have been working for herself. The general would never have approved a deal with Victor Archovy and his Belorussian drug company. The Russians and the Belarusians were barely on speaking terms, and as far as I could figure out the general would have had no control over the Archovy company.

And what about the two Bulgarian thugs? They obviously weren't taking direction from Olga any longer. Were they even working for the general? And if they were, they were too stupid to carry out any operation like beating up Archovy on their own. There had to be another of the general's agents onboard to tell the two giants what to do.

Who could it be? I hadn't a clue, but I had better work it out fast. The trip was coming to an end in a few days and I had a terrible feeling that conditions onboard were going to deteriorate rapidly.

"Man overboard! Man overboard!" came out of the PA system. The ship's horn blasted and the ship came to a halt. The cabin phone started to ring.

"Hello," I said. "Who's this?"

"It's Dr. Rosenbaum, Mr. Marcov. I was just notified that this man overboard incident might relate to the violent incidents we have been involved with. I wonder whether you would be kind enough to join me in the recovery effort."

"Of course. Where shall I meet you?"

"Meet me at the exit door on deck three."

"I'll be there."

"Thank you, Mr. Marcov."

I hurried down to deck three and met the doctor, the head of security, and the senior officer of the deck. We watched as the activity under the ship's bright lights played out and the limp body of a man was brought aboard.

"It's Dr. Petrov," Dr. Rosenbaum said as he attended the body.

"Yes, I see. So you were right that this incident and the others all seem connected," I said.

I accompanied the doctor as he and his nurses wheeled the body back to the infirmary for further examination.

Dr. Petrov was obviously dead. Besides having drowned in the choppy water around the ship, he had suffered a life-ending wound to his head and neck—almost decapitating him.

"Looks like he was caught by the propeller of a passing boat," the security officer said. "If the prop of the *Europa Star* had struck him, there wouldn't have been much left of him."

"I agree," said the doctor. "In any case, I'll prepare the body and keep him in cold storage until we can remove him from the ship for burial. I would think that the captain would want to notify his family."

"Yes, I'm sure the captain would want to do that. I'll let him know," the chief of security said.

"The captain has turned the ship around," the deck officer said. "We're returning to Venice,"

The security officer and I spoke in a corner of the infirmary.

"We have two suspicious parties who may be to blame for this," I said. "Those two large Bulgarian men: Bohdan Ivanchuk, and Andrij Babich. I've had my eye on them throughout this cruise. They also assaulted me personally."

"We'll have to bring them in for questioning tomorrow when we reach Venice," said the security officer. "No use trying to do that now. We'll have the *carabinieri* to help us in the morning, and the ship will be shut down so that no one but police authorities will be able to get on or off."

"Very well. Please give me a call in the morning when you begin the search for them," I said.

"Absolutely," the security officer said. "Good night."

"Good night," I said. I left the medical area to return to my cabin—with my hand on the butt of my revolver.

CHAPTER 19
HOMEWARD BOUND

Ruth and I hadn't slept very well, so we were up early, washed, dressed, and eating our breakfast in the cabin by ten a.m. The ship had returned to the Venice marina during the night and was securely tied to the dock. We watched from our balcony as a number of vehicles drove up to the ship's boarding platform. Most of them had "*Polizia*" in large letters on their sides. There were also two ambulances and several unmarked cars.

About a dozen uniformed carabinieri with rifles in hand marched up the boarding platform. The several attendants from the ambulances came down the platform with a stretcher on which was a well-wrapped parcel in the shape of a human body. They slid the collapsible stretcher into one of the ambulances, which immediately drove off with lights flashing and sirens blaring.

Just then, the chime on our cabin door rang. I opened the door and a ship's officer was standing there with a plastic portfolio in his hand. "May I come in, Dr. Marks? I have information about your departure arrangements."

"Of course, come in, come in," I beckoned. I introduced the officer to Ruth.

We sat on the couch and the officer placed the folder on the coffee table.

"We have arranged for you to leave from Venice tomorrow," he said. "There's a USAir flight that leaves tomorrow at four p.m. directly for Philadelphia."

"That sounds good," Ruth chimed in.

"Yes, we will drop off the tickets at your cabin door later today. Also, there will be a refund check for the part of the cruise that you missed."

"That's very kind of you," I said.

"Not at all. That's the least we can do for the inconvenience we have caused you. And because of the difficulties you've been through, we would like you to join the senior officers, and some others, at the captain's table again tonight for a farewell dinner."

"Thank you," I said.

"But I won't have any clothes to wear!" Ruth exclaimed. "They'll all be packed."

"I'm sure the captain will understand," the officer said diplomatically. "I'll leave all the departure information, except the tickets, here on the table. If you have any questions, there's a number on the front of the package that you can call."

And with that, the officer stood up, shook my hand, tipped his cap to Ruth, and departed.

"Well, I guess we should start packing," Ruth said.

"Okay," I said. "It'll give us something to do while we wait for Linda Carter."

Chapter 20
Causa Belli

The cause of war

At eleven fifteen, there was a knock at our cabin door and a jingle of our door chime. I opened the door and saw Special Agent Linda Carter looking as bright as a new copper penny. She was wearing a tan outfit today: tan jacket and tan slacks. Her blonde hair was swept back into a bun.

"Well, how are you, Linda? It's good to see you again," I said as I shook her hand.

"I'm just fine, Ham. The jet ride over was a bit rough, but I did manage to get a few hours of sleep."

"It's really good to see you, Agent Carter," Ruth said, grabbing her hands in an obviously warm greeting.

"Well, I'm here to help, officially," Linda said to both of us.

"We're very glad. We didn't know who else to turn to," Ruth said.

I ushered Linda into the cabin and sat her down on the couch. I pulled up a chair and Ruth sat next to her.

"I think I'm up to speed on the current situation. After getting the basics from you, Ham, I've spoken to the captain; the security officer; the doctor; Simeone Markov, the Bulgarian agent; and the CIA agent, whatever his name is. It appears that you are in the middle of an international drug heist. How you did it, I'll never know." Linda shook her head in disbelief.

"It was my "C" change," I said.

"Your what?"

"I'll explain later. What's the next step? Do you have a plan?" I asked.

"Well, the object of this caper appears to be the taking over of the patent for the Vanishe cream that Dr. Petrov, the dead man, invented. But whether the Russians are involved, or some other Balkan entity, is a little fuzzy right now. The plan is to round up the two Bulgarian tough guys, who seem to be the intermediaries in this deal, and squeeze them for information."

"That may not be so easy," I said. "I've seen them in action. They're quick, strong and decisive, plus sneaky."

"Yes. We all agree to those observations. The security chief and the carabinieri, along with Marcov, are making up a plan of action for their capture. I'll join them after talking to you," Linda explained.

"Well, we'll leave that to you," Ruth said.

"Yes," I agreed reluctantly. "Would you like something to drink or eat? We've got plenty of goodies here in the suite," Ruth asked.

"No thank you, Ruth. I had a good breakfast while listening to the harrowing tales from the involved parties," Linda answered.

Bang! Bang! Bang!

These were loud sounds from outside our cabin door. Ruth and I jumped up and said together, "What was that?"

"Sounded like gunshots to me," Linda said calmly. "Why don't you two stay right here while I go and investigate? After all, that's what I'm here for," Linda said with a smile as she put one hand on the door handle and the other on the handle of her weapon neatly tucked into the back of her slacks.

"I'm going with you," I said.

Now why did I say that?

"Oh, no you're not, Ham Marks! You stay right here with me," Ruth said firmly.

"Don't worry, dear. You stay here with the door locked. Don't worry about me. I have the FBI protecting me," I said with a smile.

It was a bit comical. Linda, my protector standing at five feet six, was in front of me. I was having some difficulty using her as a shield for my six-feet-two, overweight body. But out the door we went.

"Lock the door!" I shouted at Ruth as I shut the cabin door and Linda and I started down the corridor.

Chapter 21
Just Belli

War

This was the plan. The carabinieri would spread throughout the ship and try and herd the two Bulgarian bad guys onto the main deck. The security chief, the CIA man, and I would stay at different exits to the main deck in order to help out in the arrest and make sure that no innocent cruisers would wander onto the deck and into the line of fire. Agent Carter would join us at the exit closest to Dr. Marks's cabin.

I checked my weapon—again—and made sure that the laser was working properly and that I had several speed loaders ready in case I needed more than five shots.

I took a two-handed grip on my revolver and pointed it toward the deck. I stood at one side of the entrance to the main deck and made sure I could move, unimpeded, to the other side, giving me a 180-degree line of fire.

Bang! Bang! Bang!

I heard the shots but couldn't tell who was firing.

Rat-a-tat. Rat-a-tat-tat, I heard. *Uh, oh,* I thought, *that's an AK-47. Someone in this gunfight has some heavy artillery.* I carefully peeked around the doorframe and what I saw calmed me, to a degree.

The sheikh's bodyguards, hearing the shots, felt that the sheikh's life might be in danger so they fired their weapons in a haphazard pattern. Bullets were flying, and I decided to take cover until I had a target.

Suddenly I spotted one of the big Bulgarians dash behind a lifeboat suspended in its davits. He began firing his gun in all directions. It became obvious that the carabinieri had him surrounded.

Then I saw Agent Carter with Ham Marks behind her. She raised her gun to fire when—Bang! Bang!—two shots rang out, presumably from the Bulgarian. Ham went down. He had been shot. Agent Carter and I took aim at the same time and fired. My bullet followed the laser dot exactly and entered the right thigh of the big man. Carter's shot entered his left thigh, and down he went with a howl.

Carter turned to help Dr. Marks while the carabinieri officers and I ran to bind the hands of the wounded Bulgarian and drag him away. The carabinieri would place him in a van and take off quickly to the hospital to have his wounds treated. Then, if it was possible, they would take him to the local Italian prison for interrogation.

I still had one more Bulgarian giant to bring in. I reconstructed in my mind what had happened in the last few minutes. I recalled seeing a man's head pop out of one of the entryways and then pop back in. Searching my mental computer bank, I matched the man's face with another in my rogue's gallery. It was the East German engineer, Bergman. Maybe he was part of this puzzle.

Chapter 22
Takedown

I crouched as low as possible behind Linda at the entrance to the main deck. *Bang! Bang!* Two more shots rang out, and this time I felt at least one of the shots hit my left shoulder. I fell backward in pain.

Linda concentrated on returning fire. Then she turned to me. "Are you hit, Ham?" she asked anxiously.

"Yes, I think I took a bullet in my left shoulder," I said between gritted teeth.

"Okay, let's see what we can do," Linda said calmly.

She sat me up against the wall and took off my jacket and shirt. It was obvious that I had taken a round into my deltoid muscle. It was bleeding, but not profusely.

Linda examined my shoulder and said, "The bullet grazed your shoulder. There's no entry or exit wound, so there's no bullet fragment in your arm."

With that, she took out a folding pocketknife, opened it, and sliced my undershirt into several strips. She bound my arm tightly and then sat back and observed her work.

"I think you'll be all right until we can formally clean the wound, dress it, and start some antibiotics," she said.

"I'll take a tetanus shot as well," I added. "Along with some Advil."

"I'll call the doctor and have him meet you here and take you to the clinic," Linda said.

"I'll call Ruth from there—and calm her down," I said.

"Good luck with that," Linda said. "I'm going with Simeone to find the second Bulgarian. Will you be all right?"

"I'll be fine," I said. "Go, go, go!"

Off she went.

In my mind, I started trying out various excuses to tell Ruth. Suddenly I felt cold steel at the base of my neck and an accented voice said, "Get up and come vith me, and you vont get hurt. Othervise, I vill keel you right here."

"Okay, okay. I'm getting up," I agreed.

Out of the corner of my eye, I could see a man who I would have no trouble hiding behind. It was the huge second Bulgarian. He switched the gun to my back and prodded me down the corridor to the next exit door. Looking both ways, he shoved me forward across the deck and in between two lifeboats in their davits.

"Where will this get you?" I said, for reasons I still can't fathom.

"I vill trade you for escape, or I vill shoot you," the giant said.

At that point, I saw Simeone and Linda, along with three armed carabinieri. They saw me, fortunately, and didn't start to fire.

"Give it up, Bohdan! You can't get away!" Simeone shouted.

"I vill get away, or this man vill die!" the Bulgarian shouted back.

"Okay, okay. Let us work something out. No more shooting. Okay?" Simeone responded.

"Okay, I vait for you to let me get avay."

An uneasy silence settled over the deck. I figured it was worth trying a plan of my own. I certainly couldn't get into any worse trouble than I was already in.

I gradually widened my stance, and at the same time I slowly bent forward, with a groan. The big man with the gun figured I was reacting to the pain of my gunshot wound and didn't make another move.

When I was completely bent over, I reached between my legs with both hands and carried out my favorite Princeton wrestling takedown maneuver. I grabbed one of his legs below the knee and pulled as hard as I could.

The gunman gave a shout and went over backward, striking his head on the lifeboat and again on the deck. His gun went flying across the deck.

Before I could even straighten up, Linda and Simeone were on top of him with their handcuffs out.

"Ladies first," Simeone said as he helped Linda turn the giant face-down so she could cuff his wrists behind his back.

"Nice move, Doc. Where did you learn that one?" Linda asked.

"Princeton," I said. "I guess they don't teach that at Yale."

She laughed and shook her head. Simeone and the carabinieri dragged the second Bulgarian away.

Linda took me down to the medical clinic where Dr. Rosenbaum took care of me and placed my left arm in a sling.

"Now I'd better call Ruth," I said.

"Good luck," offered Dr. Rosenbaum.

"Right," I said as I picked up the shipboard phone and asked to be connected to my suite.

"Hello! Hello!" Ruth said.

"It's me, dear. Everything is fine."

"Where are you, Ham? I was worried sick with all the gunfire!"

"I'm fine. I'm in the medical clinic. I just have a scratch on my arm. I'll be up in a few minutes."

"A scratch! What does that mean? Ham Marks, you get yourself up here immediately."

And I did.

CHAPTER 23
A FAREWELL DINNER

Ruth looked great in her nonpacked outfit. I wore the jacket and tie that I had planned on wearing in the morning when we were going to leave the ship.

The captain's table was jammed full. There sat the first officer, the security officer, the officers of the deck, the doctor, Simeone Markov, Linda Carter, Dr. and Mrs. Brown, and the CIA agent formerly known as Dr. Shevenko.

Everyone was talking, and they all stopped and cheered when Ruth and I came to the table. I smiled and raised my right hand overhead, making a Joe Namath number one sign with my thumb and index finger.

My left arm, in its sling, hurt like hell, but two Advil had settled the pain somewhat. We sat and talked to everyone about the day's events and also exchanged cards so that we could communicate, or tweet as the case may be, after leaving the *Europa Star*.

I did take a glass of champagne, *for medicinal purposes,* but stuck to iced tea for the remainder of the meal. Alcohol and I don't get along too well.

The meal was, once again, superb. I can't describe each course, since I forgot to steal the menu. The chateaubriand, I can tell you, was a work of art. I even got my steak cut by the waiter who took pity on me for my sling-bound, dominant left arm.

As we finished an elaborate ice cream and cake concoction, the first officer—a slim, square-jawed Irishman—tinkled his glass with a spoon and rose with a beribboned package in his hand.

"Ladies and gentlemen," he said, "Captain Gillespie sends his sincere apologies. He had some details to attend to on shore, because of our unexpected return to Venice, so he couldn't be with us tonight. He has deputized me to make this next award in his place. Tonight we are awarding a special honor to Dr. Ham Marks. It is what we call our Chartreuse Heart award for bravery at sea."

And with a flourish, he offered the wrapped package to me. I quickly unwrapped it and came upon a glass paperweight, in the shape of a heart, with a model of the *Europa Star* mounted on it. On the glass was written "I love *Europa Star*," with a heart substituting for the word *love*. I held it up, and it glistened in the candlelight. Everyone clapped and cheered.

"Thank you very much," I said. "I'm sure that Ruth and I will never forget this trip on the *Europa Star*."

Everyone laughed and clapped again.

"And now," the first officer said, "I want to make two more presentations. These go to Dr. and Mrs. Marks and Dr. and Mrs. Brown for their cruising activities beyond the call of duty aboard the *Europa Star*."

He handed a pseudo-leather passport portfolio to Mrs. Brown and Ruth. "Inside the folder, you will each find two tickets on any cruise the *Europa Star* makes in the next year—occupying the owner's suite."

The two ladies smiled and opened the folders to show their spouses while the assembled clapped and cheered again.

At that point, the party broke up. As we were leaving the table, Linda Carter leaned over and said to Ruth and me, "Take your time going back to the suite. In about a half an hour, Simeone and I will come by and fill you in on what has happened after the battle of the *Europa Star*. Okay?"

"Fine," I said. "I can hardly wait." And off Ruth and I went, strolling arm in arm. Or I should say we were strolling *arm in sling*.

"I think I'll wait a while before I consider another cruise," Ruth said.

CHAPTER 24

FINALE

We relaxed a bit once we got back to the suite. I loosened my tie. Ruth removed her shoes and put her feet up on the couch. We barely noticed Bill O'Reilly on the TV.

Thirty minutes later, there was a *ding-dong* at the door. I opened it, and in came Linda and Simeone. Ruth put her shoes back on and ushered everyone to the dining table, where she asked if anyone wanted something to eat or drink. No takers.

Linda spoke first. "Well, folks, are you ready for the battle's aftermath? Don't worry. No Gettysburg Address."

We laughed.

"The one giant thug who Simeone and I shot recovered quickly and was delivered in a wheelchair to the Venice prison. The questioning went on for several hours. I think Simeone was the translator. Am I right, Simeone?"

"You are correct. They talked their heads off, and I translated the story into English. The notary then translated the transcript into Italian. The *ohs* and *ahs* of the carabinieri could be heard for blocks around."

"You are not going to believe who the ringleader of the merry band was," Linda teased.

"You're right. I can't wait. Was it Olga?" I guessed.

"You want to try again, or would you like to know?"

"Please tell us," Ruth begged.

"It was Captain Gillespie," said Linda.

"Captain Gillespie!" Ruth and I shouted.

"How is that possible?" Ruth asked.

Linda turned to Simeone and indicated that he should continue with the story.

"What none of you knew was that Captain Gillespie, a good Irishman, was married to a not-so-good Bulgarian lady who apparently belonged to a stable of not-so-good friends. She found out about Dr. Petrov, a Bulgarian, and his patent for Vanishe cream being on the *Europa Star*, and cooked up a plan to get it away from him and sell it to the Russians for big bucks.

"She convinced her husband, the captain, that he had been working for peanuts as a tourist ship captain and that this was his chance to strike it rich. He organized his little *band that couldn't shoot straight* around the two Bulgarian thugs, who were friends of an uncle of the captain's wife, Sofia.

"He had two cutouts who controlled the thugs and kept him out of the limelight: the engineer, Bergman, and the sommelier, Maria Mosenko.

"How exactly this group was going to convince Petrov to hand over his patent, the two thugs didn't know. Finally it was decided just to kill him and steal the patent."

"But what about Olga? Wasn't she in on this evil plot?" I asked.

"Apparently not," Linda answered. "She was just a not-so-innocent bystander."

"Her father, the general, is a powerful figure in Russia, but she apparently just fell into this messy ditch and tried to dig herself out on her own—and tragically failed," Simeone explained.

"What about Dr. Petrov's family?" Ruth asked sympathetically. "Has anyone called his wife?"

"Yes, I did," Simeone said. "She, of course, was devastated. I explained that the doctor's body was being transported back to her and that Dr. Archovy was accompanying it. The good doctor, with permission from the Belarusian authorities, volunteered to instruct Dr. Petrov's wife on how to protect the patent and how to secure the proper licensing agreement. He does have a slight ulterior motive. He is going to try and get Mrs. Petrov to agree to have his brother's company comarket Vanishe cream. She'll actually make more money that way."

"Well, I think that's very nice of Dr. Archovy, after all he went through," Ruth said.

"And that's the story," Linda said. "I think that the FBI will be happy to sign off on this series of foul deeds and let Simeone and the Bulgarian Secret Service handle it. That offers the United States another international connection that can only bring benefits to the FBI in terms of gathering information about bad guys in the world."

With that, Linda stood and said, "I'm going to stay around for another day or so. I'll clean up things with the carabinieri and then do a little shopping. I hear the Euro's down. I'll say good night to you two tonight and talk to you again after you get home."

"Thank you for everything," I said.

"Especially for getting you shot." She chuckled.

"That was my own fault," I said. "Imagine the stupidity of thinking that I could hide behind you," I countered.

"I'll say good night and good-bye also," Simeone said. "You won't have to look for my bald spot anymore."

"Your bald spot?" Ruth said.

"Sure. I saw you both staring at it all the time. After all, I do have eyes back there," Simeone said with a smile.

And with that, Simeone and Linda left the cabin.

Ruth and I wearily prepared for bed. We checked that our luggage was properly lined up outside our cabin door, lined up our clothes for going home in the morning, and fell into bed.

"You looked especially beautiful tonight, dear," I said to Ruth.

"Oh, yes? Well, thank you, but you can blame that on Vanishe cream. I used that little sample jar that Dr. Petrov gave you. Can you get me some more?" Ruth queried.

"Not unless you want me to put my life in jeopardy again," I said. "You'll just have to wait until it's released to the American market."

"Oh, okay," Ruth said reluctantly.

After a few moments of silence, I said, "I've decided to change my mind about something."

"Oh, yes. What's that?" Ruth asked.

"I'm going to change my mind and agree with the majority of folks who feel that a "C" change is the sudden change in the condition of the wind and waves at sea."

"Don't do that, dear," Ruth said sleepily. "It wouldn't be the real you."

"Okay. You're right. Good night, dear."

"Good night, Ham."

ACKNOWLEDGEMENTS

I would like to acknowledge and express my thanks to several people whose help added immeasurably to these two novellas. First, thank you to my brilliant wife, Michele, a real-life classicist, who helped with all the classic references in the books. Second, I would like to acknowledge the help of my good friend and legal eagle, Barton Haines, Esq. who helped with the legal references in book I. Next, thanks to Alex Kyourktchiev for his help with all things Bulgarian and Ukrainian. Finally, I thank Burton Stein, Esq. for his horse sense and for getting me into a real stud farm.

ABOUT THE AUTHOR

William H. Simon, MD, has practiced medicine as a board-certified orthopedic surgeon for over forty years. He is an associate professor of orthopedic surgery at the University of Pennsylvania School of Medicine. He is a fellow of the American College of Surgeons.

Dr. Simon is the author of over fifty published scientific articles, books, and videos. *Prescription Murder* is his first fictional publication.

Dr. Simon lives with his wife, Michele, in Villanova, Pennsylvania, and Jupiter, Florida.

E-mail—Docbone487@AOL.com